T0114727

ADDICTED
TO GOD AND RECOVERY

STEVEN W. MURPHY, LCDC, AADC

Acts 1:8 (NASB)
*8 but you will receive power when the Holy Spirit
has come upon you; and you shall be My witnesses
both in Jerusalem and in all Judea, and Samaria,
and as far as the remotest part of the earth.*

WESTBOW
PRESS®
A DIVISION OF THOMAS NELSON
& ZONDERVAN

WestBow Press books may be ordered through booksellers or by contacting:

WestBow Press
A Division of Thomas Nelson & Zondervan
1663 Liberty Drive
Bloomington, IN 47403
www.westbowpress.com
844-714-3454

Interior Image Credit: Brittany Rae Murphy

ISBN: 978-1-6642-8563-7 (sc)
ISBN: 978-1-6642-8564-4 (hc)
ISBN: 978-1-6642-8562-0 (e)

Library of Congress Control Number: 2022922191

Print information available on the last page.

WestBow Press rev. date: 04/12/2023

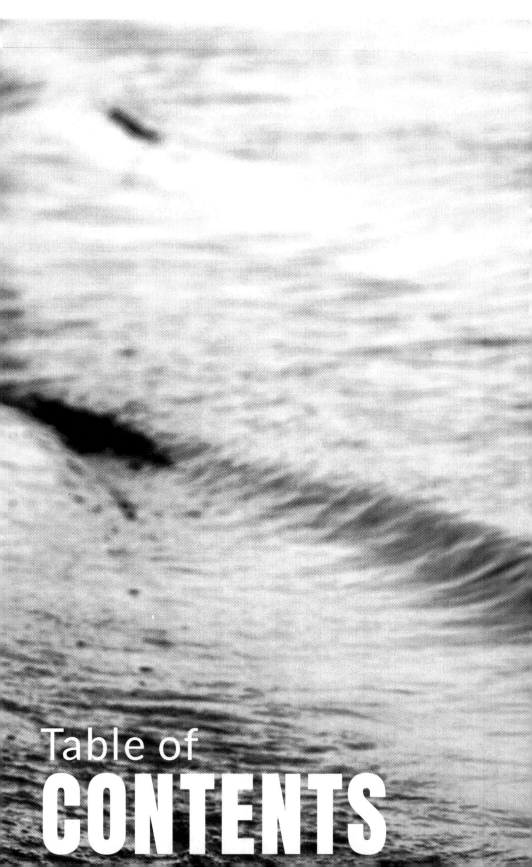

Table of
CONTENTS

INTRODUCTION

Understanding the 12-steps from a Biblical perspective.

Have you ever wondered why you do things that contradict your beliefs? In Romans 7:15, Paul is struggling with the same concept when he writes, "I don't really understand myself, for I want to do what is right, but I don't do it. Instead, I do what I hate." Paul gives us a big clue here, which is a reason why I am sharing this book with you. He "really doesn't understand" himself.

Some of you may be thinking that you don't have any problems or addictions. Many people minimize their problems and behaviors by saying that they aren't as bad as other people. If we believe we don't have any sin or issues in our life, we are deceiving ourselves, and we are calling God a liar. In Romans 3:10, Paul writes, *"As the Scriptures say, 'No one is righteous—not even one.'"* In 1 John 1:10, John tells us, *"If we claim we have not sinned, we are calling God a liar and showing that His word has no place in our hearts."*

The blessing is, _we have a way out_! In Romans 8:1-2, Paul goes on to say, *"Therefore there is now no condemnation for those who are in Christ Jesus. For the law of the Spirit of life in Christ, Jesus has set you free from the law of sin and of death."* We don't have to keep feeling shame if we stop the behavior and reconcile the damage because God has paid all of our debts. The power of Jesus Christ overpowers the laws of sin and death.

If we stop and think about it, many of our problems are a result of the denial of an issue, minimizing a problematic event, keeping a secret, or developing a variety of unhealthy behaviors. These start to occur because we are trying to reduce pain in our lives or the lives of others. Most of us develop unhealthy habits. It starts by doing something that seems exciting, illegal, and not too immoral. Many of us have consumed alcohol underage, smoked pot, tried drugs, had sex outside of marriage, gambled, manipulated others, been victims of other people, lost control of our anger, or lived in fear. There are many other activities we may have participated in and habits we wanted to stop but have had difficulty doing so. When we start practicing crazy behaviors, doing illegal, immoral, or unethical things, we become separated from the majority of people we interact with and start interacting with people who do the same things that we do.

Unhealthy behaviors separate us from God. We don't like to look at them or talk about them, and our practices continue to overpower us in our lives and negatively impact others. We try to stop them daily however, we keep losing control. We ask God for help, but He doesn't seem to respond, or we don't like the answers we receive. We refuse help and continue to affect those around us while our shame continues to grow.

If you have experienced these problems in any area, you are normal.

If you've tried to control them with various solutions but have been unsuccessful, you are human.

If you ask God for help, but it seems like you don't receive an answer, you may be blinded to God's solutions.

If you have tried what God said, but it didn't work, you may have stopped before the miracle happened.

This book will help you see the patterns, stop the behaviors you can stop, get help for the behaviors you can't stop, and use the resources God has provided through Scriptures, 12-step recovery, and Christian living. This book is not written to twist the Scriptures or the word of God, but rather how to use inspired processes to help us overcome sin and destructive behaviors in our lives.

God has many paths to salvation and each of our testimonies shows our own personal adventure with God. We wait on Him to guide us and sometimes he guides us by leading us to fellowships that can help us overcome harmful behaviors in our lives. If God doesn't heal us immediately when we pray, should we continue in our sinful behaviors? Should we try to find resources that will help us? Does God want us to self-destruct or to move forward in a healing process? I hope this book is an inspired resource that helps you overcome every obstacle that blocks your way to a relationship with your Creator.

FOUNDATIONS

My Family & Early Recovery

Reasons for Writing

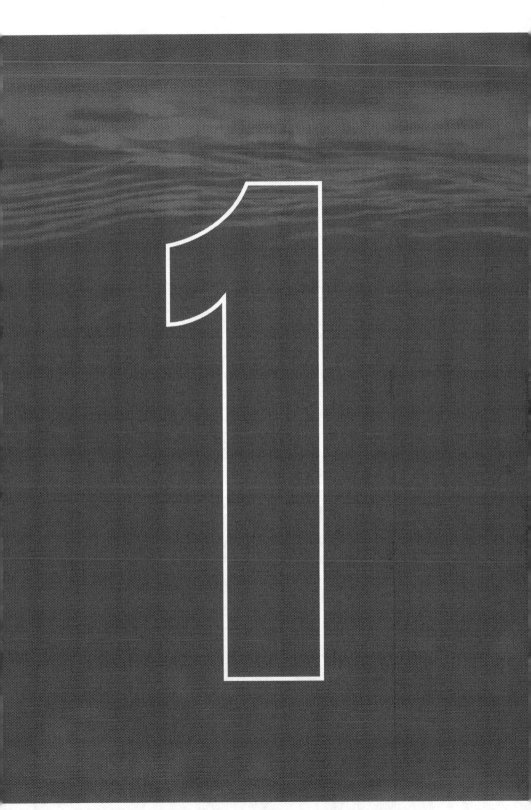

chapter one
FOUNDATIONS

My Family & Early Recovery

I was raised in a family that had problems with alcohol, but alcohol seemed customary to me. My parents encouraged us to participate in the scouting activities, while my alcoholic father was a supportive parent of the activities. When I was 10 years old, I wasn't aware of his drinking, but my mother was. When she confided in me about dad's drinking, I felt a lot of pressure to help mom to figure out ways to get dad to stop. He was unsuccessful at 12-step meetings for five years until he checked into a 28-day drug rehab. As soon as my mother found peace in a family 12-step group, and my father maintained recovery, my brother and I started using alcohol and drugs. Our parents tried to get us to go to church, but I felt so guilty for what I had done on Saturday night that I could not sit in the pews on Sunday morning. Within five years, I was drinking 6 to 24 beers every day. By my senior year in high school, I was drinking anything with a high percentage of alcohol in it; my favorite being an entire pint of rum.

I did try to keep my breakfast drinking "healthy" by adding orange juice to my rum in the morning on the way to school. I was smoking pot every day, and my motto my senior year was "at least one joint a day." Before "wake and bake" (smoking marijuana for breakfast) became popular, we smoked a bowl of "WEEDies" for breakfast. I used methamphetamines, LSD, painkillers, Valium, inhalants... anything I could get my hands on. My A/B average started dropping. I was head photographer for the yearbook and newspaper and had opportunities to go to college, but I didn't care. I was more focused on getting high and doing it every day, all day. I was arrested three times, lost friends, lost girlfriends, lost jobs, lost money, lost faith, lost my reputation... well, actually developed a reputation, but not the one I wanted. Because of the excessive use of the chemicals, I did things I never thought I would do. The shame and guilt turned into depression and hopelessness. I believed that God hated my guts, and I felt my lifestyle was more in line with the devil and sometimes gave him credit for who I was. I stole cars, broke into vehicles, broke into houses, and when I was caught, I wondered why I had so much bad luck. I didn't need to steal; I just would rather spend someone else's money than my own.

I attempted numerous ways to control my problems. I tried stopping on my own three times, saw therapists, doctors, tried different types of 12-step meetings, tried to only score from "trustworthy" drug dealers, but I kept getting caught and problems continued to increase. I cannot remember if I ever prayed for help from Jesus or God; I am sure I did. Nothing seemed to help. I eventually felt so depressed after numerous bad experiences in life that I tried to kill myself by overdosing on pills two times and cutting my wrists one time. I scared many people. Not because my life was permeated with evil, but because I was so self-destructive. As I look back now, my life was filled with darkness. I had become unethical, immoral, selfish, self-righteous to cover my pain, and lost all of my values. My family eventually encouraged me to seek residential treatment. I knew I needed to stop, but I only wanted to slow down or cut back.

By this time in my life, my father had attained four years of sobriety by attending 12-step meetings meetings. My mother had been going to family 12-step groups for at least four years. My grandfather and my grandmother had at least 20 years sober in 12-step recovery from alcohol and in the family group, respectively. The week before graduation, I had maintained seven days without using alcohol or drugs. The abstinence did not occur by my efforts or abilities rather by my parents who were vigilant in their determination to make sure I stayed sober. They were constantly transporting me everywhere I needed to go and kept me at home whenever possible. On graduation night, I relapsed by drinking and smoking with one of my best friends. My father was proud of me for graduating from high school but more grateful that I was still alive. He shook my hand, congratulated me, and then realized I had relapsed. He told me, "You have a choice. You can either move out tonight because you broke your promise when you said you wouldn't use alcohol and drug anymore, or you can check into treatment." Since I didn't have any significant plans on where to live, and I had not followed through on any of my college opportunities, I reluctantly decided to choose the treatment option. Somehow, he had arranged for me to be admitted to residential treatment the night I graduated from high school. I was immediately transported to the hospital and checked into a 28-day program.

I resisted recovery and hoped that they would teach me how to drink socially, but I soon discovered recovery was all or nothing. I continued to believe I was going to be able to control my alcohol and drug use but gradually began to realize it wasn't possible. During my second week of treatment, I was still in denial. I thought I was too young to be addicted. I didn't do my homework and had plans to drink less once I left the hospital. A counselor saw through my evasive behaviors and asked me, "You have tried staying sober on your own, seen good counselors, therapists, and doctors; now you are in residential treatment. Your parents and grandparents have been in recovery and worked 12-step programs. Steve, can you stay sober without working a 12-step program?"

I said, "I know this one guy –"

He said, "Stop! I'm not talking about one guy, I'm talking about you. Can you stay sober without working a 12-step program?"

I said, "Well, some people –"

He said, "Stop! I'm not talking about some people; I'm talking about you. Your father has four years sober in recovery. Your grandfather has 20 years sober in recovery. Your mother and grandmother are both involved in 12-step family groups. Can you stay sober without working a 12-step program?"

This was the first time I actually reflected on my unsuccessful efforts to stop. I pondered the concept and then quietly said, "No. I can't."

He told me to go to my room, complete my Step 1 homework I had been avoiding (because I didn't want to look at myself), and that we would talk about it the next day. From that point forward, I focused on recovery. A week later (day 21 of residential treatment), my therapist asked if I was ready to graduate in 7 days, and I told her, "No, I just realized last week that I was an alcoholic and an addict. I need another week." I graduated from the treatment center two weeks later, with 35 days sober, and have been sober ever since. I am sober by God's grace, from following the instructions of wise people who have been willing to share their time and personal experiences about recovery, and living a more godly life. Early Recovery started with me finally admitting I had a problem, then utilizing the resources of people who have already had recovery experience and following their paths. They shared that they had to rely upon God, which I learned how to do. They told me, "If you don't know how to pray at least say this: 'God help me stay clean and sober today' and at the end of the day say: 'Thank you for letting me stay clean and sober today.'"

> **"I RESISTED RECOVERY AND HOPED THAT THEY WOULD TEACH ME HOW TO DRINK SOCIALLY, BUT I SOON DISCOVERED RECOVERY WAS ALL OR NOTHING."**

CHAPTER ONE

I learned to read recovery material, pray, confess, be honest, follow the path of the 12-steps, meditate, follow my mentor/sponsor, socialize with sober people, and attend 12-step meetings. I haven't been able to do this perfectly but have been reasonably consistent for 40 years. So far. It's only by God's grace and being obedient to His gentle guiding hand that I am here.

Over the years, I have seen many people find new and better lives through recovery. I would never trade my life experiences for anything. I was deeply ashamed and humiliated by my addiction. I was ashamed of early recovery and having to be "in recovery," but now I realize it is an asset. It is a gift I have been given. It was and is a second chance to make something of myself and an opportunity to help others find solutions. My God is a God of second chances. He helped me to find a new life in recovery, and then He helped me find salvation. Nothing I did, condemned myself for, or thought about could ever separate me from His love and opportunity for redemption. I have been given many opportunities: to live on this earth, escape addiction, find recovery, find salvation, and have a life filled with blessings and opportunities even through the hardships.

Many have chosen various paths of spirituality; some have followed the faith of their fathers, while others have walked away from their faith. Some subscribe to the spirituality found in recovery, which is good however, it is not all that we need.

I saw my father and mother return to the church. They used the 12-steps to enhance their spiritual walk and reconnected to Jesus through the fellowship of their Baptist church. I saw my grandfather and grandmother resume their faith. And after my daughter was born, I started to feel that the spirituality of 12-step recovery was not enough. When she was three months old, my wife and I returned to the church.

There have been times in my recovery when I've felt so distant from God that I must walk into an empty sanctuary, physically drop down to my knees at the foot of the cross, ask God to forgive me, remove the barrier. Some of these occasions have been a result of my behaviors & shortcomings; others are just a longing for a deeper relationship with Jesus Christ. In some instances, I don't know why I'm so far away from God, but I find reassurance in knowing He is always there. Sometimes my ego requires that I go where He resides. I know He lives in me, and He is in my home, yet I find a stronger connection when I go to God's House.

I'm Writing This Book For Many Reasons

#1: My hope is that this book would bridge the gap between people in recovery and the church. I believe people in recovery can set aside their religious biases, find a church and develop a deeper relationship with God. I hope and pray that they realize countless fathers of our faith and the founders of recovery have had meaningful spiritual relationships with God, and know He is real. I would hope they could find a way not only to read the AA Big Book, the NA basic text, or any other 12-step program's "big book," but to understand the **BIG** Big Book-***the Bible***.

I believe that God inspires many recovery books, but it's essential to read the original book inspired by God. The founders of AA read the Runners Bible daily and primarily focused on the Sermon on the Mount in the book of Matthew, the entire book of James, and 1 Corinthians 13:4-8 (Love is...). Many people in recovery don't want to hear that the foundations of our redemption are based on Christian scriptures. Twelve-step programs keep their recovery programs "non-sectarian" to allow people to avoid the bias of conflicting religions, denominations, or spiritual beliefs. They offer recovery from horribly destructive diseases to anyone open to spiritual concepts, so they can at least start on the path to healing.

#2: This book is to help people in the church understand that 12-step recovery is inspired. It has its roots in Judeo-Christian beliefs. Many people who have found recovery after they left a church fellowship have stated the fellowship in recovery "is how the church should be." The understanding in recovery is that we are all powerless over our addictive/compulsive/sinful behaviors, and as a result of living a destructive existence, we have damaged many aspects of our lives. No one is any better or worse than anyone else in recovery.

#3: This book is in memory of a dear friend who led a recovery ministry. Yvonne Peterson did many amazing things in her life. She was a counselor, a healer, an LVN, a Christian, and a warrior. She passed away in December 2003 from complications with the flu. During my time working with her, we participated in Celebrate Recovery at our church. We saw how John Baker (with the support of Rick Warren) had developed the Christian 12-step recovery concept of Celebrate Recovery.

If you look at the 12-steps and the scriptural parallels utilized by Addicts for Christ, Alcoholics Victorious, and Celebrate Recovery, you notice that they are scattered throughout the Bible. I have always been curious if the 12-steps were in order anywhere throughout the Scriptures. After Yvonne Peterson passed away, God gave me a Scripture to help encourage the 20 stunned mourning leaders of Celebrate Recovery. We continued to carry a recovery message at our church. I shared the Scripture in an email to all of the leaders. I had an opportunity to share my testimony at another church that had started a Celebrate Recovery. Halfway through my testimony, I shared the Scripture that God had given me with the church leaders and realized, "These are the 12-steps!".

I have shared the Scriptures in Second Peter with people over the years, and it has helped many people see the 12-steps from a biblical perspective. We will discuss this more in chapter 3.

#4: It removed my fear of carrying a message from God. I am sharing the scriptures that have been revealed to me. They confirmed the 12-steps are the core of a spiritual program of recovery that was validated by Scripture. I don't believe anyone has ever indicated where the 12-steps came from. I have searched the Internet and read many books trying to find if anyone has ever found the path and pattern of the 12-steps within 1 or 2 chapters of any book in the Bible. I know recovery works, but I also wanted to be sure that once I resumed my Christian walk that I wouldn't do anything to minimize my relationship with my Savior. I did not want to idolize 12-step recovery over God.

#5: I have seen so many people struggling to see God or find solutions to their many problems. We have begun to rely heavily on science, technology, and man's wisdom that we have ignored the eternal wisdom of God that always has relevance, whether it's yesterday, today, or tomorrow. There are many who are struggling with anxiety (fear) and are not aware that the solution to fear is faith. Many who are overcompensating for their shame and humiliation. As a result, we become arrogant and egotistical instead of accepting weaknesses with humility and finding real strength. Fear and pride will always be our downfall. These unhealthy emotions are evident throughout the Scriptures, spiritual teachings, and recovery writings.

Recovery is not just for drug addicts and alcoholics! The Oxford English definition of recovery is: "the action or process of regaining possession or control of something stolen or lost." Whether we lost our way, or we allowed addiction/addictive lifestyles to steal from us, there is a ***process to regain possession***!

Other issues, such as unresolved or ongoing depression, grief, hurt, neglect, and abuse, overtake our lives. We can fall into traps with drugs, alcohol, medications, food (chemical addictions), behaviors like sex, gambling, video games (process addictions), and other practices. These behaviors separate us from God, remove our trust, diminish our faith, and cause us immeasurable pain (physical or emotional). When seeking solutions to these problems, where should we search in the Scriptures, that would tell us how to stop. Where would we suggest another person start reading? When people told me scriptures, I didn't understand what God's words meant. I felt so condemned and separate from God. If I am an alcoholic, will reading the first chapter of Genesis get me sober? What if I read the last chapter of the book of Revelation? John 1? Romans 8? From these readings, I might learn about the beginning of everything, the end of everything, who created everything and the path to eternal life, God's love or salvation, but they didn't keep me on track to stop my addictions and sinful habits. I prayed for God's help, but He had an alternate route for me. Some addicts need a step-by-step process to develop understanding to find a solution.

APPLICATION

Finding Our Purpose

Holistic Healing

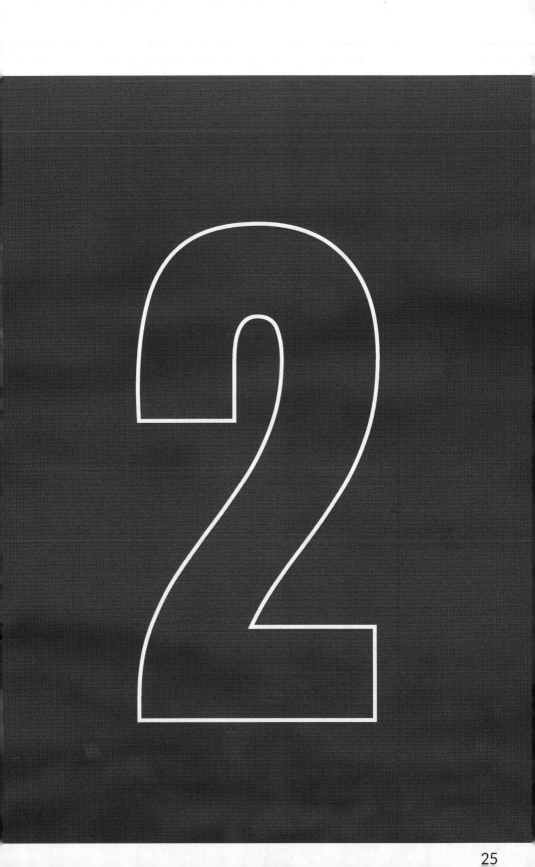

chapter two

APPLICATION

Finding Our Purpose

God revealed 12 chapters in the scriptures in the Old to the New Testament that embody the concepts of the 12-steps. In this book, we will identify **one** chapter that confirms this path. We will explore the lives of those who followed the Word of God by a pattern of the 12-steps vs. those who neglected everything they knew fueled by an addictive impulse that did just as much damage to their lives thousands of years ago as it still does to us today.

Many people in recovery have returned to a walk of faith and worship as they practiced recovery principles and have overcome their anger at God as a result of working the 12-steps. One of the greatest blessings I've been able to receive is seeing lives drastically changed for the better. I see minds restored, bodies healed, families and communities repaired. I see fellowship, the love of Christ, peace, and deep meaning return or develop for the first time. Lives are touched by not just knowing about God, but removing the wreckage and blockage from our lives and truly getting to know God.

One day, many years ago, I spoke to several people in a recovery group who had been practicing the 12-steps. I asked them, "What is the greatest gift you have experienced as a result of leaving your addictions and living this new sober life?" In one way or another, they all stated, "I now know God" or "I know God better".

Ken Freeman, a fantastic Christian evangelist, whose teachings bring the scriptures to life, shared this remarkable insight based on Philippians 3:13 New Living Translation (NLT)

"13 No, dear brothers and sisters, I have not achieved it,[perfection] but I focus on this one thing: Forgetting the past and looking forward to what lies ahead,..."

Ken proceeded to teach:

"The enemy says look back;
Comparison says look around;
Shame says look down;
Jesus says look ahead."

A man in our married couples group at church asked me, "Where did you get such strong faith?" He and his wife grew up in church, went to Christian universities, and were very active in their Christian walk. He stated he was reading a book about a Christian missionary who prayed to God before departing for his first mission. The missionary told God to slay him if his ministry ever did damage to the gospel of Christ. The Christian husband stated he was afraid to pray that prayer for fear that God might slay him. I told him, "I had to have that faith in God and stay focused on the recovery process, or I was going to die."

Have you ever wanted a closer relationship with God?

Have you ever wanted to feel His presence?

Have you prayed and asked for answers, but He didn't answer?

Have you ever wanted to speak with Him, but didn't feel worthy?

He wants to hear from us and speak with us.

Sometimes in the silence, He is waiting for us to do the last thing He told us to do.

Sometimes the answer is "No."

Sometimes we feel as though we are not worthy to speak with Him or to receive His blessings or even to utter His name.

This book is _not_ written to teach us how to get what we want from God, but instead for us to fulfill God's purposes. It's about how to clear away the wreckage of our past, change our attitudes, increase our faith, and find what God wants us to "do" to be obedient to Him. Our problem is we don't honestly know God. We know the stories. David and Goliath. Noah's Ark, Samson, and Delilah, Jesus born in Bethlehem, Jesus dying at Calvary and His resurrection, but we don't know who God truly is or why He does what He does. Some of our hesitations are fears, presuming embarrassment of being viewed as a religious or recovery fanatic, and the overwhelming task of doing what we don't want to do.

"I don't really understand myself, for I want to do what is right, but I don't do it. Instead, I do what I hate." Romans 7:15

God is the great physician. The mighty counselor, but we don't want to get too close because we are afraid He will reject us. He might ask us to do things we are uncomfortable doing. Our unresolved pain holds us back. Our issues block us from truly being all that God created us to be.

How do we get to know who God is? How will we learn what He hopes for our lives? Do we know what He can do? It is by reading, understanding, and living the Scriptures. It is by asking God, seeking healing deliverance by God, and meeting God that we begin to understand how our unhealthy habits or sinful behaviors impede our relationship with Him. When we find recovery from our old lives, we start sharing our experiences and hope, which encourages others to find Him.

Some of these paragraphs are written from the perspective of "we"; others are written from a personal perspective. This book is written in the context of "we." This book is written with the understanding that we are all sinners **AND** all are children of God. We all have to decide if we are going to be active members in the family of God, rebellious children, or outside observers. We need help, and the Scriptures are instructions from God to improve our lives. The 12-steps provide us with a path to find the healing that God makes available to us to follow through His word. Most people in recovery or who are seeking recovery have been too proud, too fearful, too depressed, or too unworthy to seek God in church. Some of us did seek help in the church but the church was unable to provide an approach that we could understand.

> *"13 For merely listening to the law doesn't make us right with God. It is obeying the law that makes us right in His sight. 14 Even Gentiles, who do not have God's written law, show that they know His law when they instinctively obey it, even without having heard it."* Romans 2: 13-14

Fulfilling God's purposes may not seem to be what we desire, but OUR sinful desires remove us from fulfilling God's purposes. Our purpose is to glorify Him, which in turn will richly bless us and help others. He will help us if we listen to Him. He will help us if we ask Him. He is always with us, always watching out for us, and gives us everything we have. He is above us, beside us, and within us. He is the Father, the Son, and the Holy Spirit. He is **everything** we will need, but we will have to weed our garden and get rid of everything that prevents us from growing into who He created us to be.

Our relationship with God changes as we grow. If we learned about God as small children, we were taught to pray before meals, before bedtime, pray for others, and pray when we were sick. As we started attending school, we prayed for help with tests, prayed for boyfriends or girlfriends, things we would like to have, and prayed to make problems go away. When some of those things didn't happen, we wondered why God would not answer _all_ of our prayers.

As we grew into our teen years, we started rebelling. We started having intellectual conversations about the existence of God that were influenced by our education. Science and philosophy made faith seem even more illogical. But peer pressure eventually provided an excuse to distance ourselves from God. When we had problems, our difficulties seemed too big for God to resolve, or, at least, it seemed He did not care to fix them. As we began to have doubts about His existence, He became a fairytale, or a myth, or a crutch for some people, but not for us. Some teenagers stayed active in the church in church activities; some did it for the fellowship, some for the intimacy in relationships and the possibility of losing the dating relationship if we didn't go through the motions necessary to keep the relationship. We eventually stopped our participation in church and believed that we could continue to have a relationship or at least be good. We made the classic comments of, "I don't have to read the Bible." "I don't have to go to church to have a relationship with God." These statements are accurate; however, we lose the accountability to the fellowship of other believers who would encourage us and hold us responsible for our actions. We lost the mentoring of the Sunday school teacher. We forgot the history lessons from the Bible and the wisdom of the Creator of the universe. We explored our interests, daily life distracted us, and we quit making time to read the Scriptures. We didn't have time to pray, and gradually we forgot lessons we had learned. We started practicing behaviors that contradicted God's ways and discounted what we knew as children.

> **WE WILL HAVE TO WEED OUR GARDEN AND GET RID OF EVERYTHING THAT PREVENTS US FROM GROWING.**

Losses, bad decisions, unanswered prayers, and injustices resulted in resentment towards humanity and God. We started to search for meaning in other activities, spiritual practices, unethical behaviors, and sometimes illegal deeds. We justified our actions by blaming God, using God, or eventually denying that God exists. Some of us will shut God out altogether. We contemplated returning to our Christian ways, but we didn't want to have to suffer the way some of "them" do. We don't want to be ridiculed for our beliefs or live life by such stringent rules. We want life to be easy, but it has its difficulties whether we have faith or we don't.

There comes a day when we realize we are damaged, and there is nothing on earth that can fix that brokenness. For some of us, our relationships have become so deprived of human qualities such as compassion and civility, that it would take a miracle to repair them. Or we encounter a situation in which there seems to be no way out. We experience losses, life changes, personal attacks, abuse, or injustices and wonder why God would allow these things to happen.

Eventually, we realize God is not responsible for how we live, we are.

We have all been dishonest at some point in our lives, some of us daily.

We avoided making the changes we needed to do.

We have avoided a relationship with God for fear of what He may ask us to do.

We have all sinned. All of us sin every day and fall short of the glory of God.

Whatever it is that causes us to be dishonest or disobedient, transitions to a neglect of our responsibilities. When we are disobedient, we sin against God, hurt others, or damage ourselves, which becomes a barrier to living a full life. Whatever blocks us from being honest and doing what is right, will hinder us from a relationship with our Higher Power. Confessing our sins to God (1 John 1: 9), coming clean to others (James 5:16), or admitting to ourselves (Romans 3:23), opens the door to the healing process. However, repeating the behaviors without changing our lives impedes the recovery process and our relationship with God.

Think about this. If we are not living the way we know we are supposed to live by God's standards, do we subconsciously understand that we are misbehaving but asking God to reward us? It seems that the longer we live a destructive lifestyle, the more our thoughts become self-deceptive, bordering on insanity.

People who have never had a problem with addictive behaviors: gambling, shopping, sex, or chemical addictions to food, alcohol, or drugs usually approach people who suffer from these behaviors by encouraging them to "be strong," "be determined" or "just stop, as I did." Most people who are addicted to chemicals or behaviors have already attempted these measures. We try herbal remedies, prescription medications, over-the-counter drugs, home remedies, self-determination, willpower, staying busy, counseling, hypnosis, prayer, or any other "quick fix" that we can find.

What we haven't examined is how long it took us to develop these dysfunctional behaviors. We aren't considering how they have slowly evolved in our lives over the years and the gradual modifications we made in our lives.

- The physical rituals or needs.

- How our thinking has adapted to an addictive lifestyle of justification and defensiveness.

- The intense feelings that are connected to the thought of no longer having the behavior.

- How our spirituality has become idolatry by worshiping and praying for what our flesh desires.

- The network of friends we have found that endorse our harmful practices or the fact that we have lost our friends.

Our desire to feel good has altered our perceptions, eventually resulting in our addictive lifestyles. We believe if we can rid our lives of the problem behavior, then everything will be fine. We want God to clean up our problems however, the bad habits we have picked up along the way will take time to resolve. God can remove it immediately, and He can also provide us with a way out.

*"¹³The temptations in your life are no different from what others experience. And God is faithful. He will not allow the temptation to be more than you can stand. When you are tempted, **He will show you a way out** so that you can endure."* 1 Corinthians 10:13

I pray that this book blesses your life. I pray for you to receive a path and pattern to live by when you have nowhere else to go. I believe that you will find peace, kindness, the fruit of the spirit, and real faith. From a relationship with Jesus and the filling of the Holy Spirit, you will positively influence the lives of everyone around you. I pray that the lives you change through the work you do faithfully for God will provide you with an eternal relationship with our Father in Heaven, and I look forward to seeing you there. Amen.

Holistic Healing

The problem with addiction is that it is a holistic illness. It's an illness that involves the mind, the body, the spirit, the heart, and relationships, which requires holistic healing. If we just physically stop drugs, alcohol, gambling, sex, controlling others, anger, fear, depression, cutting, self-mutilation, overeating, anorexia, bulimia, or any other unhealthy habits, we are only taking care of a fraction of the problem. Physically stopping the behavior does not address how we have developed a habit of overcoming the lack of intellectual coping skills, emotional responses, social isolation, or spiritual practices. Addictions cripple addicts. Growth in all these areas is underdeveloped. Instead of responding appropriately to situations, we emotionally overreact. Those who have difficulty socializing take a few drinks, and they can talk to anyone. As time progresses and their habits worsen, they avoid or lose almost every relationship. They will eventually avoid spirituality. After all, it reminds them of what they are doing wrong and will participate in their addiction because it empowers them and helps them feel like a god.

We are a five-part being. We are physical, emotional, intellectual, spiritual, and social. We love our addictive habits and behaviors and commit everything we are to them. We fall in love with the physical and emotional gratification, we try to avoid thinking about our obsession, we ignore our conscience, values, morals, and ethics, and our social circle shrinks as a result of our compulsive lifestyle. The solution to this unhealthy devotion is found in Scriptures and recovery. It is best replaced with a strong commitment to God. We see this five-part total commitment to God in Luke 10:27

"27'You must love the Lord your God with all your heart, all your soul, all your strength, and all your mind.' And, 'Love your neighbor as yourself.'"

Most people don't like it when God is introduced to the equation. However, if He is the Creator of the universe and everything we know, why did He create us? If we had remained committed to our faith, would our life decisions be better or worse? If we had sought to do what is right instead of making ourselves feel good through earthly desires, would we be contributing more to society? Or would we be taking from our communities the way our negative behaviors cause us to do?

Another way to look at the degree our sins or addictions impact our life is how they become so overwhelming that they prevent growth in every aspect of our being. Let's discuss steroids for a moment. With most addictions, we physically neglect ourselves (unless we're doing steroids, then we overdo our physical well-being at the cost of our intellect = because we know steroid use is bad for us).

Why do we seek steroids?

To bulk up? Did we do this for _physical_ gratification? Ego? To _feel_ better about ourselves?

To _impress_ others? Using steroids will improve our physical stature, but at what cost? Low self-esteem?

To win competitions? Did we cheat when we use steroids secretly? Did we get them from a legitimate source?

Are we trying to be something that God did not create us to be?

Are we not satisfied with what God gave us? Do we think we can do better than God?

Are we willing to pay the price? Don't we realize that people will notice?

Steroids cause emotional overreactions with anger. We don't socialize with people who blame us for using, and we try to hide the fact that we are on steroids. Spiritually we are corrupting our body, attaining an illegal substance, affecting our ability to procreate, and doing damage to internal organs. <u>We are self-medicating to accomplish a specific effect. We are willing to practice behavior that will cause damage in the long run. We forget the fact that we are not medical professionals (usually) who are self-administering or self-medicating mind and body-altering chemicals. We think our behavior is good, but it only impresses a small population. When considering that we are in bodybuilding or athletic competitions with others who don't use steroids, we ignore the fact that we have cheated ourselves and others by disqualifying ourselves from an honorable challenge</u>.

I could explain ten other addictions all with similar correlations. There are numerous books written about addictions and recovery, however this book is an effort to find a spiritual connection for holistic healing. I have often read the Scriptures in verses throughout the Bible and wondered how do I do the things that God wants me to do? An example can be found in 2 Peter 1:4-7.

"4 And because of His glory and excellence, He has given us great and precious promises. These are the promises that enable you to share His divine nature and escape the world's corruption caused by human desires. 5 In view of all this, make every effort to respond to God's promises. Supplement your faith with a generous provision of moral excellence, and moral excellence with knowledge, 6 and knowledge with self-control, and self-control with patient endurance, and patient endurance with godliness, 7 and godliness with brotherly affection, and brotherly affection with love for everyone."

Through Peter, God gives us this beautiful chain of events that will occur. I don't know how to make them happen, but I can guess. <u>Everyone will have a different spiritual experience</u>, but this is what I've gathered from verse 4...

- I trust God and know that He only has the best hopes for me. I know some of His promises and that by accepting Christ, I will be able to share in His divine nature.

- If I go to church and study the word, I will escape the corruption caused by human desires. I can speculate that as I continue to respond to God's promises, my life will get better.

But how do I supplement my faith with a generous provision of moral excellence? And how do I specifically improve my moral excellence by knowledge? And if I know, how do I practice self-control. I know a lot of people who have knowledge but have poor self-control. If I practice self-control, I understand that I will have to patiently endure the changes and how my behaviors and lack of self-control negatively impact others. As I patiently endure the changes, I become more of what God wants me to be by being devout and a godly person. As I become a better person, I developed closer bonds with those who are my brothers and sisters, and then eventually, I learned how to practice these behaviors with everyone.

But again, the question is, how do I transition through this transformation? Does it naturally occur? If I just read the Bible or go to church or attend Sunday school? If I am in a twelve-step recovery, do I keep attending 12-step meetings, find a mentor, follow the 12-step path, or read the book/instruction manual for the 12-steps?

I started praying about implementing God's word in my life. Not as a way to "do works" or for self-glorification, but to do my part by surrendering, accepting, self-examination, correcting, and disciplining my life. I was trying to find the balance between seeking God's will for my life but also taking action. I have learned that studying God's word gives me insight. Reading daily meditations helps me prepare for the day. Fellowship increases my strength and hope.

12-STEPS

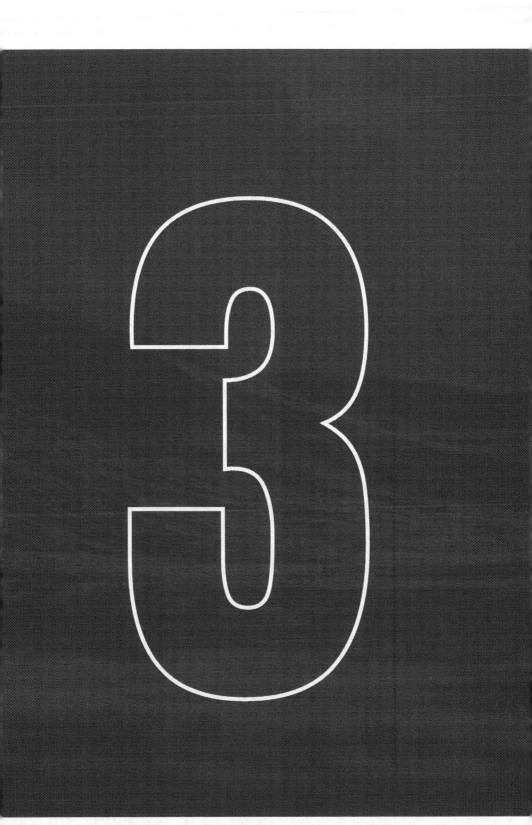

chapter three
GETTING TO KNOW THE 12-STEPS

What are the 12-Steps?

Think about this. If we have a problem in our lives and we finally admit it, we start the process of healing by exposing the issue to the light. We usually pray for a solution or seek people who have overcome the same type of problem we're experiencing. We pray to God for the strength to keep this problem out of our lives. We may journal or document insights about similar behaviors in our past, discuss them with somebody we trust, and then pray that our problems are removed. We may feel the need to rectify these past indiscretions we have inflicted on others as a result of the joy of overcoming problems and reducing the emotional burden that we have been carrying. Then we continue to watch for those behaviors and correct them as soon as they occur. Practicing corrective actions improves our ability to pray (speak to God) and meditate (listen to God) since our burdens, guilt, and shame have been lifted and as a result of all these wonderful experiences and overcoming problems, we gladly help others and share what we have learned. This paragraph embodies steps 1 through 12 in their simplest form.

Listed below are the 12-steps, excluding the specific habits (alcohol, food, sex, anger, gambling, spending, other people, abuse, pornography, emotions, etc.) with Biblical comparisons utilized by Christian 12-step groups (Celebrate Recovery, etc.).

Step 1 - We admitted we were powerless over _____—that our lives had become unmanageable.

"I know that nothing good lives in me, that is, in my sinful nature. For I have the desire to do what is good, but I cannot carry it out." Romans 7:18

Step 2 - Came to believe that a Power greater than ourselves could restore us to sanity.

"For it is God who works in you to will and to act according to His good purpose." Philippians 2:13

Step 3 - Made a decision to turn our will and our lives over to the care of God as we understood Him.

"Therefore, I urge you, brothers, in view of God's mercy, to offer your bodies as living sacrifices, holy and pleasing to God–this is your spiritual act of worship." Romans 12:1

Step 4 - Made a searching and fearless moral inventory of ourselves.

"Let us examine our ways and test them, and let us return to the LORD." Lamentations 3:40

Step 5 - Admitted to God, to ourselves, and to another human being the exact nature of our wrongs.

"Therefore confess your sins to each other and pray for each other so that you may be healed." James 5:16a

Step 6 - Were entirely ready to have God remove all these defects of character.

"Humble yourselves before the Lord, and He will lift you up." James 4:10

Step 7 - Humbly asked Him to remove our shortcomings.
"If we confess our sins, He is faithful and just and will forgive us our sins and purify us from all unrighteousness." 1 John 1:9

Step 8 - Made a list of all persons we had harmed, and became willing to make amends to them all.

"Do to others as you would have them do to you." Luke 6:31

Step 9 - Made direct amends to such people wherever possible, except when to do so would injure them or others.

"Therefore, if you are offering your gift at the altar and there remember that your brother has something against you, leave your gift there in front of the altar. First go and be reconciled to your brother; then come and offer your gift." Matthew 5:23-24

Step 10 - Continued to take personal inventory, and when we were wrong, promptly admitted it.

"So, if you think you are standing firm, be careful that you don't fall." 1 Corinthians 10:12

Step 11 - Sought through prayer and meditation to improve our conscious contact with God as we understood Him, praying only for knowledge of His will for us and the power to carry that out.

"Let the Word of Christ dwell in you richly." Colossians 3:16a

Step 12 - Having had a spiritual awakening as the result of these steps, we tried to carry this message to others, and to practice these principles in all our affairs.

"Brothers, if someone is caught in a sin, you who are spiritual should restore him gently. But watch yourself, or you also may be tempted." Galatians 6:1

The Anti 12-Steps

On the other hand, when we have a problem, we usually don't want to admit it. We hide it, we avoid it, and we try to protect it from others, which causes more senseless behaviors. We are angry at God for "giving us" the problem and don't trust Him to help us. We don't want to talk to anyone about it, we just want it to go away, or we want to be normal again. We don't want to write about it, look at it or think about it. We don't want to talk to anyone else about it, and we don't know how to get rid of it. We try to avoid the people we have hurt by our behaviors. We defend our past actions, and we don't want to admit that we were wrong because life is just too hard. We don't seek guidance from our Higher Power to do the right things, but we only pray to get us out of trouble or fix the wrong things we have done. We continue to negatively impact our lives and the lives of others by our behaviors. These practices would be the anti-12-steps.

Michael Visger developed the anti-12-steps in 1996. As a counselor, he took each of the 12-steps and twisted them to the extreme opposite. In doing so, he revealed that the behaviors that naturally occur as a result of our addictions and self-destructive behaviors contrast the solutions that remove us from our addictive behaviors. He has taken the 12-steps and rewritten different versions for addicts, overeaters, sexual behaviors, codependency, work-aholics, hoarding, survivors of incest, codependency, debt, emotions, criminal lifestyles, nicotine, and video games. Again, the 12-steps could be modified to any sinful behavior. A finding at Celebrate Recovery indicates that only 1/3 of the people that attend 12-step meetings have alcohol and drug problems; the remaining two-thirds have other issues.

CHAPTER THREE

Let's look at the anti-12-steps and the (12-steps).

1. I declared that I have total control over breaking God's law, and that I can completely manage my life and still get away with sin.

(We admitted we were powerless over our sinful behaviors, and that our lives had become unmanageable.)

2. Came to know that I need no one and that breaking God's law helps me maintain my happiness and sanity.

(Came to believe that a Power greater than ourselves could restore us to sanity.)

3. Made a decision to harness the benefits (as I understand them) of any sin I want to commit.

(Made a decision to turn our will and our lives over to the care of God, as we understood Him.)

4. Made a searching and fearless moral inventory of all others.

(Made a searching and fearless moral inventory of ourselves.)

5. Admitted to no one, including myself, any of my wrongs, no matter how evident.

(Admitted to God, to ourselves, and to another human being the exact nature of our wrongs.)

6. I became entirely ready to defend, excuse, and justify my actions, using personal attacks on others (if necessary), and to minimize any mistake I make.

(Were entirely ready to have God remove all these defects of character.)

7. Boldly declare that I have no shortcomings (while secretly believing that anything bad I ever did could not be forgiven).

(Humbly asked Him to remove our shortcomings.)

8. Made a list of all persons that had (or that I thought had) harmed me and searched for opportunities to collect on those debts.

(Made a list of all persons we had harmed, and became willing to make amends to them all.)

9. Collected whatever I felt that I was owed whenever possible, even though doing so may cause injury or harm to someone else.

(Made direct amends to such people wherever possible, except when to do so would injure them or others.)

10. I continued to take an inventory of others' wrongs against me and promptly collected on them when possible.

(Continued to take personal inventory and when we were wrong promptly admitted it.)

11. Sought through experimentation, expert opinions, partying, and the advice of my sinning friends, a better, consequence-free lifestyle. I search only for more knowledge of how and what is fun and profitable to do, and the means to do so without consequences.

(Sought through prayer and meditation to improve our conscious contact with God as we understood Him, praying only for knowledge of His will for us and the power to carry that out.)

12. Having an enjoyable experience from not getting caught, I tried to carry this message to other suffering God-fearing people to lead them to practice these principles in all their affairs with me.

(Having had a spiritual awakening as the result of these steps, we tried to carry this message to others, and to practice these principles in all our affairs.)

When Mr. Visger originally wrote the anti-12-steps, he asked those who knew the 12-steps to consider, "If the anti-12-steps are what people do in their addictions (or compulsive behaviors), wouldn't it be logical to work the 12-steps to overcome the behaviors?"

The Beauty of the 12-Steps

The 12-steps help us find solutions to a problem. The First Step asks us to identify our attempts to control our behavior and the negative impact our dependencies have had on our lives. Steps 2-12 are the answers to the problems we found in Step 1.

In **Step 1**, we explore the truth of our inability to control destructive behaviors. Whether it is a chemical addiction (alcohol, drugs, food, etc.) or a process addiction (gambling, driving fast, power, work, cutting, etc.) or it is a person that we love, seek to control, or controls us. We conclude that we can't control it, are out of control, or have lost control. We may have tried to quit our behaviors, cut back, slow down, limit frequency, amounts, time, avoid places, avoid people only to find that we repeatedly falter.

Step 1 also asks us to explore what parts of our lives have been negatively impacted. We must honestly assess if our behaviors have had a negative impact at work, our occupations, careers, endeavors, goals, schooling, our interactions with our parents, siblings, children, distant relatives, friends, spouses, or coworkers.

Has it caused painful emotions such as depression, shame, fear, resentment, or remorse?

Has it caused us to neglect or abuse ourselves physically, hygienically, medically, psychologically, sexually to lose who we are?

Have we sought God or a spiritual experience, only to be further away from Him?

Have we denied Him?

Have we traded eternal life in Heaven and our purpose on earth for a false sensation that feels heavenly and demanded fulfillment of our purposes?

CHAPTER THREE

Is our behavior costing us financially?

Do we feel like we are losing ground rather than gaining?

Are we blaming someone else for all of our problems when the real perpetrator has been looking back at us from the mirror the whole time?

> " [23] *For if you listen to the word and don't obey, it is like glancing at your face in a mirror.* [24] *You see yourself, walk away, and forget what you look like.* [25] *But if you look carefully into the perfect law that sets you free, and if you do what it says and don't forget what you heard, then God will bless you for doing it.*" James 1:23-25

Only by revealing our inability to heal will we seek healing and ask God to help us. Only by knowing what we have lost will we be willing to change our lives. We have revealed the problem, let's start finding the solutions.

Step 2 helps us understand that we need something or someone greater than ourselves to resolve this problem. Everyone in recovery immediately looks to God for this solution, but God provides us with a history of humans who have failed and succeeded based on their self-determination or God-centered focus. God will provide a power greater than ourselves in the form of a professional, a group, a book, a new way of life, and even a connection to God through Scripture, radio broadcasts, and sermons. For most addicts, God is the first AND last. He is the first choice because we are hoping for a painless resolution and an easy answer. He is the last choice because we have repeatedly asked Him to make our problems go away but to no avail. The "Powers greater than ourselves" mentioned in Step 2 also includes our sponsor/mentor/elder, the steps, the Scriptures, recovery books, relying on God, and fellowshipping with other believers/recovering people. We should have a sponsor by Step 2 to recap Step 1 and guide us through the 12-Steps.

Step 3 helps us realize that we need to surrender to a Higher Power to help us live better lives and make better decisions by being empowered by God. Many people early on in recovery don't want to surrender their lives because they feel they have lost control. They feel they have lost their will to choose and damaged their lives with their past destructive behaviors. They cannot see how surrendering their will and lives to God will be any better. In fact, due to the shame, resentment, and fear that most addicts experience, it is difficult to surrender to a being they have never seen. Some fear that God will retaliate (punish or neglect them) and be vengeful towards them for the many things that they have done while in their addictive lifestyle. Some feel they will be forced into a lifetime of spiritual servitude which will result in them working hard and never having fun again. However, we have all found that **until we surrender** our lives and our wills over to God, we will continue to fail.

" GOD WANTS US TO HELP ALL THE CAPTIVES KNOW THERE IS A WAY OUT AND THERE IS FREEDOM."

They think, "Why should I surrender my life to God? I have already surrendered my life to my addiction and I don't want to be a servant to God like I was a slave to addiction." They don't realize the fact that they will either be a **servant to God** or a **servant to addiction**. The beauty of our Christian walk is that God is like a ruler who purchases slaves and then sets them free. Most addicts have had to live in fear and can't imagine a kind loving God.

"[28]Then Jesus said, 'Come to me, all of you who are weary and carry heavy burdens, and I will give you rest. [29]Take my yoke upon you. Let me teach you because I am humble and gentle at heart, and you will find rest for your souls. [30]For my yoke is easy to bear, and the burden I give you is light.'" Matthew 11:28-30

*"¹And so, dear brothers and sisters, I plead with you to **give your bodies** to God because of all He has done for you. Let them be a living and holy sacrifice—the kind He will find acceptable. This is truly the way to worship him. ²Don't copy the behavior and customs of this world, but let God transform you into a new person by changing the way you think. Then you will learn to know **God's will** for you, which is good and pleasing and perfect."* Romans 12:1-2

As we begin to know Jesus Christ truly, our discussions reveal that God never attaches strings and makes us puppets. He cuts strings, breaks chains, sets captives free, and wants us to share our recovery with others. God wants us to help all the captives know there is a way out and there is freedom. The only being that attaches strings is Satan. He is the one that wants us to be chained, bound, and dead. He is the one who revels in our pain and thrives on us spreading our addictions to others.

Step 4 asks us to look at our lives from many different angles. Step 4 is difficult. It takes time and deep self-examination. It also comes at exactly the right time. After we surrender our lives and our will to God, we feel a sense of peace. Many people in recovery do the "recovery 3 step". They think, "I found a solution to my problem, I have new friends and I have God; I'm good, I don't need any more help." The problem that arises is: the enemy or the disease starts talking to us about our past.

"Remember all those people who hurt you? You need to get them back!" (Resentments)

"Remember all those people you hurt? They'll never forgive you!" (Harm we have perpetrated on others/shame)

"Remember how many times you've tried to stop before? You'll never stop. You'll fail again." (Fears)

"It looks like nobody loves you. You don't even love yourself. You don't even know what love is!" (Intimacy)

This is why we are asked in Step 4, to write about our resentments, harm done to others, fears, sex, and intimacy. I have often heard the saying:

"When the enemy (Satan/the disease) reminds us of our past, remind him of his future." - Saint Teresa of Avila

Another saying, *"Every saint has a past, every sinner has a future."* - Oscar Wilde

Overcoming our past glorifies God and becomes part of our testimony to encourage others on the path to knowing God better. Dwelling in the pain results in decay, destruction, an unfulfilled life, and eventually, death.

"³¹Get rid of all bitterness, rage, anger, harsh words, and slander, as well as all types of evil behavior. ³²Instead, be kind to each other, tenderhearted, forgiving one another, just as God through Christ has forgiven you." Ephesians 4:31-32

Step 5 asks us to share our negative behaviors with God, ourselves, and another human being. This disclosure teaches us that we must confess to God because He can heal us and remove our sins.

"¹⁶Confess your sins to each other and pray for each other so that you may be healed. The earnest prayer of a righteous person has great power and produces wonderful results." James 5:16

Acknowledging behaviors to another human being helps us to see that we are very similar to one another in our sinful behaviors, and his prayers for us will bless us.

"⁹But if we confess our sins to Him, He is faithful and just to forgive us our sins and to cleanse us from all wickedness." 1 John 1: 9

This concept of confession has been used by clergy and people struggling with sin for thousands of years. The healing process and experience of letting these resentments, fears, harm done to others, clarifying love and intimacy will open our eyes to a remarkable world of faith, love, forgiveness, humility, wisdom, and strength.

Step 6 helps us to identify behaviors, actions, and attitudes that we need to be "willing" to release from our lives to acquire a better existence and consider replacing it with the "fruit of the Spirit." Step 6 is where we decide if we are <u>willing</u> to stop being dishonest. Are we ready to reduce our pride, stop self-destructive behaviors, ease our shame? Will we examine how fears, anxieties, and worries have driven us to unhealthy activities and impulsive reactions? We decide if we are willing to give up the negative and start living in the positive.

Look at Galatians 5. Wouldn't we all be willing to trade out the lusts of the flesh... *"Sexual immorality, impurity, lustful pleasures, idolatry, sorcery, hostility, quarreling, jealousy, outbursts of anger, selfish ambition, dissension, division, envy, drunkenness, wild parties, and other sins like these"*...for the fruit of the spirit?

*"The Holy Spirit produces this kind of fruit in our lives: love, joy, peace, patience, kindness, goodness, faithfulness, gentleness, and self-control. **There is no law against these things**!"*

Think about that last sentence. "There is no law against these things!" All the other lusts of the flesh have criminal statutes in almost every country in the world.

"[12]Restore to me the joy of your salvation, and make me willing to obey you." Psalm 51:12

After writing our inventory, reviewing the causes, and exploring our defects of character, we can be restored to joy by obeying God, getting rid of our worries, forgiving those who have hurt us, and become willing to change our behaviors that hurt others. Doing these things will bring us so much closer to the life that God wants us to have.

I met a man who had been through treatment 15 times. I asked him if he had picked treatment centers and programs that were incompetent or provided poor service. He responded, "Some were better than others, some were worse than others." I then asked why he had been unable to stay healthy in his recovery. He simply stated, "I didn't follow instructions." Some people think they are smarter than their doctors, some believe they are more experienced than their therapists, and some people think they are above God's help.

In **Step 7**, we ask God to remove our shortcomings. Because of our experience in recovery and participation in the fellowship, we have discovered there are some behaviors we cannot stop on our own. Hopefully, by this time, most of us have learned that God, through recovery, has helped stop certain behaviors, actions, and attitudes, and we are responsible for replacing the vacancy of the defects with assets. We have learned positive recovery behaviors or have started adopting a spiritual, Christian lifestyle. God can help us root out the problem. Still, it is our responsibility to plant healthy, effective behaviors throughout our lifestyle and consistently take care to improve and nurture these behaviors.

"¹⁰Create in me a clean heart, O God. Renew a loyal spirit within me." Psalm 51: 10

This is one of the only ways that we will be able to resolve our past is by asking God to help us be better people today. However, we can't be God's vision unless we ask God to clean up our hearts and our past.

When God removes our shortcomings and we start practicing new and better behaviors, we consider the people that were negatively impacted by our undesirable behaviors and prepare to clean up the wreckage of our past.

Working the steps to this point leads us to **Step 8**. We make a list of people we had harmed, list the damaging behaviors we have had towards others, and find in our hearts a willingness to seek forgiveness for our past indiscretions. Correcting our injuries inflicted on others will help us remove the shame, fears, and resentments to restore relationships.

Step 9 urges us to interact directly with people we've hurt through our past behaviors, addictions, fears, anger, unhealthy pride, and unwholesome concepts of intimacy. The step urges us to make amends. Amends are not just apologies. We would ask people to consider amendments to the Constitution. The amendments to the constitution are not apologies, but "improvements" to the document, not an apology for the document. They may rectify aspects of the text that were not considered in its development or modify the material to reflect situations that have changed. One issue that differentiates apologies from amends is that an apology is usually a postponement of the problem until we do it again. "Asking for forgiveness without changing our behavior is a lie." As we get closer to God, we change our behaviors for the better.

Step 9 also takes time and patience. We have found that we need to prepare for the event with our sponsors. Sponsors help us check our motives, develop our discussion, wait for the right opportunity, and ask God to help us with the words we will use. We discuss the approach with our sponsor to ensure that we are not blaming people for our problems. Most of the people we need to make amends to are readily available, but in many cases, we may need to seek out people that we have not seen for many years or live far away. We must be patient for the right opportunity to present itself and also endure the outcome, whatever the result may be.

"²³So if you are offering your gift at the altar and there remember that your brother has something against you, ²⁴ leave your gift there before the altar and go. First, be reconciled to your brother, and then come and offer your gift." Matthew 5:23-24

Matthew 5:23 is a message from God to prompt us to get rid of everything that interferes with giving to God. If we stop and think about it for a moment, every time that we give our gift at the altar, and we are thinking of people we have harmed, are we giving our gift to the one we have offended because we are thinking of them more than we are thinking of God. Is it a form of restitution or contrition to the one who is wounded by our transgressions instead of what is supposed to be given joyfully to God for our gratitude? Cleaning up our past allows us to be present and focused on the blessings of today. Are we hoping that God will clean up our trespasses so we don't have to? I have made the mistake of waiting for God to magically fix my relationships. However, God is not codependent. He encourages me to clean up my messes, grow up, practice humility and heal what I need to heal.

In **Step 10**, we evaluate our conduct daily and make every effort to avoid repeating negative behaviors discovered in our inventories by identifying them, resolving them, amending them, and sincerely changing them. All we are doing when we ask for unrepentant forgiveness in a disingenuous manner of making a temporary stop to our problematic behavior that we will resume because we have not made a sincere effort to stop by doing what Jesus would do.

"So stop telling lies. Let us tell our neighbors the truth, for we are all parts of the same body." Ephesians 4:25

This Scripture in Ephesians reminds us that every little lie, dishonesty or omission affects our community, our relationship with God, negatively impacts others, and weakens our thought of ourselves.

In **Step 11**, we continue to speak to God through prayer and listen for His guidance through meditation in the hope of living a better, more positive life and serving Him.

CHAPTER THREE

"May the words of my mouth and the meditation of my heart be pleasing to you, O LORD, my rock and my redeemer." Psalm 19:14

This Psalm and this step remind us that God's consistency, strength and mercy only come by seeking Jesus, speaking to God, and focusing on the Holy Spirit within us.

In **Step 12**, we take all of the positive behaviors learned, practice them each day, and share the lifestyle to help other people find the recovery we have been so freely given.

In its simplest form, we take Steps 1 through 12 by evaluating: if you have a problem, admit it, find help, ask God for more help, examine your ways, seek help from others, ask God for help to remove really difficult problems, clean up your wreckage of the past, be aware of negative actions, change your behavior daily if they resurface, seek God's will and help others.

"But you will receive power when the Holy Spirit comes upon you. And you will be my witnesses, telling people about me everywhere-in Jerusalem, throughout Judea, in Samaria, and to the ends of the earth." Acts 1: 8

Some people carry the message naturally; all people need God's help. Sharing the good news is the last message and instruction we received from Jesus.

These 12-steps are *so successful* that OVER 180 other 12-step groups have come into existence.

Taking Action

One disclaimer we want to make is that these scriptures will not define every aspect of recovery. They aren't going to indicate: talk to your sponsor 2-4 times per week, go to 90 meetings in 90 days, or read the recovery text (for whatever 12-step program you may need). What they will do is identify negative aspects of not working the steps, behaviors we need to avoid, or positive aspects of following God's word, applying Scripture to our lives, and help us use the steps to put God's instruction into action. Our recovery is individualized by what we hear in 12-step meetings, big book studies, or testimonies. Our Christian walk is personalized by what we hear in church during a sermon, Bible studies, and mentors. Sometimes the preacher/priest/pastor will discuss a book of the Bible, a chapter, a sentence, or the significance of a word. We learn what is being implied, but we don't know how to put it into action.

Throughout this book, we will be discussing chapters of Scripture that capture the concepts of the 12-steps AND how using the 12-steps can help us accomplish our part of the works needed to develop or maintain our faith. The scriptures in these chapters are going to present the positive and negative aspects of human behavior and God's directions for a better life. Some of the verses will indicate what we should do about a step and others will indicate what we should not do. When God says, "don't bear false witness", isn't He also saying, "don't lie," "tell the truth," "be honest," "quit being dishonest," "don't lie in front of others," "don't lie in court," "tell the truth in all that you do"? This results in the same context in many different ways.

People in recovery, pondering the foundation for the origin of the 12-steps, have attributed their beginning to the concepts taken from the Oxford Group. We have found that just as God wants us to understand the Old Testament so we can have a better understanding of the New Testament, we also need to understand the history of 12 step programs. Not just for how we live today, but to understand what has and has not worked in the past. Christianity can lead to abstinence. Our next level of growth was not just stopping the destructive behaviors in our lives, but living a godly life through recovery that resulted in significant internal discoveries in sobriety. We learn to correlate them to our experience concluding with the hope of knowing God better. Understanding the history of Christianity helps us understand what God wants, how to stop sin, and overcome this world by helping others and following in the steps of Jesus Christ. Understanding recovery helps us to understand what the founders experienced in the development of the program; the need for fellowship and that recovery is only acquired by living it and giving it away. Testimonies of Christians and recovery "stories" help us to learn lessons from the Scriptures when we read about the people of the Old Testament and the demonstrations of God's hand in the lives of addicts in recovery materials. We see the good and bad recorded in the Scriptures and, hopefully, learn lessons of what to do and not to do. Reading the Old and New Testament

"WE HAVE TO REALIZE THERE IS NOT ENOUGH FOOD OR SEX OR DRUGS OR MONEY OR ANYTHING IN THE WORLD TO FILL THE GOD-SHAPED HOLE IN OUR SOUL."

and understanding what it is revealing will occur on many different levels as we study the word. For some of us, it is just a story of people who lived thousands of years ago.

The Bible is a series of books that are historical, poetic, spiritual, prophetic, wisdom-filled, philosophical, practical, intimate, and healing. We are encouraged through a series of lives touched by God and events from the past, which teaches us about our foundation and our origins. Scripture describes obedience as well as consequences and lawful principles that eventually evolve to grace. Interspersed through all the books and stories is the image of a Savior. We see a Father who desires a loving relationship with His children, a son who sacrifices His life, and a Holy Spirit who fills us with wisdom and a connection to the Trinity. The promises of God and the Savior begin in Genesis and culminate in the book of Revelation. Jesus detailed these promises to the two travelers on the road to Emmaus in Luke 24:27

"27Then Jesus took them through the writings of Moses and all the prophets, explaining from all the Scriptures the things concerning himself."

People who have had problems with addictions to alcohol, drugs, food, sex, other people, gambling, hoarding possessions, self-mutilation, or any other behavior that human beings find pleasurable (or use to relieve pain), will use them to distract themselves from their problems, pain, boredom, and lives instead of using healthy, spiritual or practical resources. We will engage in these behaviors to avoid looking at ourselves. We do them to fill the emptiness in our soul, but we have to realize there is not enough food or sex or drugs or money or anything in the world to fill the God-shaped hole in our soul.

We have also seen the parallels between a recovery lifestyle and a Christian lifestyle. In both lifestyles, we pray, we meditate, and we study the good book in church or the recovery books of our recovery program in twelve-step recovery. We can either follow the path of the 10 Commandments, 8 Beatitudes, or some other Scripture that we value in the church. In recovery, we follow the 12-steps of recovery. In the church, we have spiritual mentors or leaders; in the 12-steps we have sponsors. We meet for Sunday school or Bible studies. In recovery, we attend meetings or big book studies. We have spiritual ceremonies and words that we say in church just as we have a format for our meetings in recovery.

The reason for this book is not just to demonstrate the parallels/similarities of our Christian walk to our recovery experience, but to point out the need for people to pursue God's word as an important part of their recovery.

In our walk through recovery, we have developed a fairly simple understanding of the 12-steps. Just as we can find significant depth in the words of Jesus and the writings of the apostles, there is significant depth to the words of the recovery books. Some recovering people have tried to resume their Christian walk by attending church spirituality. This resulted in condemnation and doubt. Many Congregations don't understand people who have had addictions. As discussed earlier, recovering people felt separated from a Christian fellowship because of their un-Christian behaviors. They have felt condemnation from God because of their interpretation of scriptures. Fortunate people in recovery have returned to safe churches and found a deeper relationship in the church which provided them with fulfilled lives.

On the other hand, the recovery fellowships have a deep, significant understanding of the needs of a person healing from destructive behaviors. Some of us have found we need recovery **AND** church to find spiritual fulfillment. **Beware** of telling a recovering person who has been attending a church, that they don't need 12-step recovery groups anymore. There is a level of accountability necessary to sustain sobriety. The decision to attend church and recovery is a decision between the recovering person and God. Not to say that 12-step recovery groups are penance for those who have avoided God while in their addiction but sometimes it appears that recovering people have to atone twice as hard to clean up the years of decadence. We are not implying "works" over grace, however, some of us are called to be a part of a ministry that requires intense self-examination with accountability. Think about the ministry that Paul was called to do. How many of us would be willing to be scourged, shipwrecked, stoned to death, and imprisoned for our faith? How many of us would leave our homes and travel the country or to other countries to carry the message of their Lord? Many recovering people understand the sacrifice that is necessary to keep our "walk" consistent, but also the importance of "giving it away" to keep it.

One reason we recommend leaving the recovering person active in a 12-step fellowship AND church, is the equipping and filling the cup in preparation for working with newcomers.

An example would be if a person attended a 12 step group and church, and that person appeared to be emotionally distressed at church, the church fellowship or friends of this recovering person would approach him and ask, "Is everything okay?" To which the addict would respond, "Yes, everything is alright." The church members may offer if the recovering person needs any help or needs to talk, they should call them or let them know. This lack of disclosure on the part of the recovering addict may be the downfall of the addict by denying their struggles/problems to appear positive and spiritual. Recovering people have a desire to be normal. The desire to avoid exposure, confrontation, and continuing to hide from their truths is a heavy yoke for anyone to bear and often leads to relapse. This is similar to seeking solutions to our medical conditions on the Internet instead of setting and attending an appointment with a physician.

On the other hand, if a recovering person who attends church was at a 12-step meeting and appeared emotionally distressed, another person in the recovery fellowship would ask if they were okay. If they responded the same way by saying, "Yes, everything is alright." The recovering person would look at them and say "Okay, I'll ask you one more time. Are you doing okay? Because you don't look okay, you look like you are about to do something destructive." At this point, the recovering person would either get angry and defensive (unhealthy fear/unhealthy pride) OR become uncomfortable and realize that the emotional distress they are experiencing needs to be disclosed and is evident to others. It is evident in their demeanor, and someone else in recovery has seen that emotional distress before (usually in the mirror). We need to be open and honest about our problems. An addict can usually see distress in another addict. Many of us are blessed to have people who will lovingly confront us and restore us to "right-thinking". My life has been saved and restored numerous times by people who have lovingly or bluntly questioned me when I was hiding my emotional distress.

We have also seen addicts find Christ by returning to church and eventually being told by members of the church fellowship that they need to stop attending 12-step meetings. The problem is: God has set these recovering addicts to minister to people in 12 step groups and the church. We have seen people who have left the recovery ministry with over a decade of sobriety, relapse and return to an addictive style within less than 12 months. People have often stated "You are a new creation in Christ. Why do you keep saying that you are a recovering addict?" We just want to make it clear that almost every single addict, no matter what their addiction, has asked that God remove the addiction from their lives. We will gladly profess and glorify God when He has delivered us from a problem. Some of us have been blessed by the removal of sinful behavior, while others have had to "walk the path" of recovery.

We find an example of this in Paul's life when he discusses, in 2 Corinthians 12, that he has prayed three times for God to remove a thorn from his flesh. What Paul found is God gives him strength each day when he surrenders his weakness to Christ. Even though Paul (through Christ) healed many and knew that God could heal him, he accepted that God had a special plan for him that did not include recovery from his "thorn."

People in recovery who have prayed for addictions to be removed. One man smoked two packs a day starting from the moment he woke up. Before he rolled out of bed, he would light a cigarette to help him wake up. One evening he asked God to remove his desire to smoke. He stood up from the prayer and knew that God had removed the addiction from his life. He immediately threw away his lighter, cigarettes, and ashtrays. He states the next morning he woke up, read his devotional, prepared to go to work, ate breakfast, and an hour later he is leaving his home for work, checking his pockets wondering "What is missing? What am I forgetting?" As he is patting his pockets he immediately realizes, "Oh yeah, I quit smoking last night!" We have found that God removes some of our defects with ease, but with others He asks us to walk on a journey of discovery and recovery with Him.

"People who conceal their sins will not prosper, but if they confess and turn from them, they will receive mercy." Proverbs 28:13

Conflicts Between Our Christian and Recovery Walk

We have found that people avoid the 12-steps because they are uncomfortable. After all, it is hard work, because it doesn't immediately fix their problems. Just like scriptural principles, 12-step recovery principles have to be applied, practiced daily, and incorporated into our daily lives. The question we would ask is: are we willing to do the work it takes to get rid of our addictions and problems? Or do we prefer to repeat the same lifestyle that brought us to these crossroads?

Some of the things we attempted were:

- We attended one 12-step meeting per month when we were drinking every day. (Not enough medicine/recovery)

- We went to church once a month but never read scriptures, prayed, or participated in a fellowship. (Hoped God would do all the work)

- We went to therapy under the influence of mind-altering chemicals and thought the therapist was ineffective. Some of us don't remember any of the therapy sessions because we were so intoxicated, we doubted the effectiveness of the treatment or felt unworthy. (Needed more help than we wanted to admit)

- We read self-help books that encouraged us to interact with others, but we didn't want to expose our shame to other people. (Too proud)

- We tried to change our emotions and moods however, the chemicals, behaviors, or temptations kept "calling to us". (Temptations and lack of support)

- We tried to move to other cities to leave our problems behind; however, they were with us everywhere we went. (Geographic cures)

- We attempted to find a romantic relationship and someone that could "save us," but unfortunately, we brought them down also. (Looking for the wrong type of love)

- We tried these and hundreds more to avoid the full effect of recovery, and the full power of healing from Jesus. We did not want to be led by the Holy Spirit and were fearful of what God would ask from us if we surrendered our lives to Him. Each compulsive behavior has its own list of attempts to control.

In recovery, we are urged to be Honest (step 1), Open-minded (step 2), and Willing (step 3). This is HOW we stay sober.

This is the Serenity Prayer:

God grant me the serenity
to accept the things I cannot change, (step 1)
courage to change the things I can, (step 2)
and wisdom to know the difference. (step 3)

The long version of the serenity prayer continues to say:

Living one day at a time,
Enjoying one moment at a time,
Accepting hardship as the pathway to peace.
Taking, as Jesus did, this sinful world as it is,
Not as I would have it.
Trusting that He will make all things right
if I surrender to His will.
That I may be reasonably happy in this life,
And supremely happy with Him forever in the next.
Amen.

Christianity and Twelve-step recovery are incredible blessings to our society and world. Sometimes we need other insights and perceptions to help us find solutions. Twelve-step recovery helps people overcome destructive behaviors, but most of all, it could bring us to a level of spiritual understanding that we would have never had or been able to find because of earthly pleasures. I can't even begin to explain what Christianity has done for the world, but one thing that helped me understand was Henry Blackaby's Experiencing God. In the book, he states that "Christianity is not just a religion, or just rules and teachings but about a relationship with a loving God."

After a period of recovery, we will find that the philosophy and lifestyle of 12-steps are life-altering, but recovery alone is not enough. It was modeled after Christian teachings and has been modified to numerous other religions.

A very intelligent young man sat in my office one day discussing spirituality.

He asked, "So you're saying I should practice a religion."

I responded by saying religion and spirituality were the foundation of recovery.

He then asked, "Should I be Christian, Buddhist, Muslim, Hindu, or what?"

I responded by asking him which spirituality aligned most with his belief system.

He stated, "I guess Christianity. So, should I be Catholic, Protestant, Lutheran, Methodist, Baptist, or Episcopal?"

I asked which one aligned most of his spiritual beliefs.

He responded, "I guess it would be Baptist.

Should I be Southern Baptist, Primitive Baptist, Free Will Baptist, First Baptist, or what?"

I asked him which one most aligned with his beliefs, and he stated, "I guess Southern Baptist."

Then I asked him, "What profession do you want to practice when you grow up?"

He said he wanted to be a doctor.

I asked him if he wanted to be an orthodontist, optometrist, neurologist, or cardiologist.

He said, "I guess I want to be a cardiologist."

I asked him if he wanted to be a surgeon, do research, or do testing.

He said, "I'd like to be a surgeon."

I asked him if he wanted to specialize with infants, children, or adults? He said he was not sure.

Just as this young man would seek mentors to explore the gift that God gave him to be a healer, he also would need to find spiritual mentors to determine his place on God's earth. Similarly, as we have to determine the course of our profession and understand how we are gifted, we also need to explore our spirituality and what separates us from, or reconnects us to God.

Please pray before you read, hear with an open mind, and allow your heart to be healed. May God bless you and help you to find a deeper relationship with Him than you ever imagined through your faith **and** your works. May you find the discipline and peace, with God's help, to overcome any addiction or bad habit, historical unforgiveness, or any behavior that blocks your relationship with Jesus Christ.

"[16]All Scripture is inspired by God and is useful to teach us what is true and to make us realize what is wrong in our lives. It corrects us when we are wrong and teaches us to do what is right." 2 Timothy 3: 16

PETER

Why is Peter Important?

2nd Peter

Steps One-Twelve

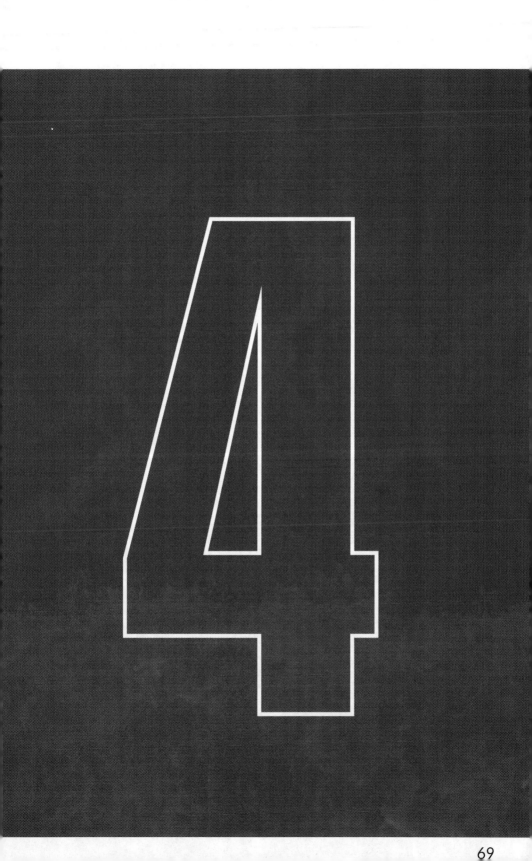

chapter four

PETER

So, Why is Peter Important?

The first section of Scripture I have found that embodies the concept of the 12-steps is in 2nd Peter.

Why is Peter significant as a disciple, and a leader of the 1st-century church?

- Because he was the first disciple and saw all the other disciples chosen. He was a witness from the beginning of Christ's ministry. (Matthew 4:18-20)

- Because Peter was the only disciple to have a family member (mother-in-law) healed by Jesus. (Matthew 8:14-15)

- Because he saw all of Jesus's miracles. (Matthew 14:13-21)

- Because he participated in Jesus's miracles. (Matthew 14:22-31)

- Because he was the only disciple to walk on water. (Matthew 14:22-31)

- Because God revealed to Peter that Jesus was the Messiah. (Matthew 16:13-19)

- Because he bragged about his commitment to Christ and had to be humbled. (Matthew 26:30-35)

- Because Peter thought Jesus should not die on the cross and knew better than God. Jesus rebuked him and called him "a stumbling block". (Matthew 16:23)

- Because he said he would never deny Christ, but fear caused him to lie. (It causes all of us to lie.) (Matthew 26:30-35)

- Because he was the defender of Jesus and drew his sword on the Roman and Temple guards, cutting off the guard's ear, but Jesus healed the soldier. (John 18:10, Luke 22:50-51)

- Because Jesus called for Peter and the disciples immediately after He was resurrected. (Mark 16:6-7)

- Because Satan targeted Peter and the other disciples. (Luke 22:31)

- Because Jesus forgave Peter and the disciples. (John 20:21)

- Because despite Peter's denial Jesus still wanted him to carry the message to the world. (John 20:21)

- Because Jesus selected Peter of all the disciples to "take care of my sheep." (John 21:15-17)

- Because Peter was the rock that Jesus was going to build the church with. (Matthew 16:18-19)

- Because Peter boldly proclaimed Jesus to the people of Jerusalem. (Acts 2:22-41)

- Because Peter was not afraid of anyone anymore. He faced his past, overcame and accepted God's prompting to change the world. (Acts 4:5-12)

- Because Peter was the 1st disciple called to minister to the Gentiles and the 1st disciple to share the good news, baptize Cornelius (Roman soldier) and his family who were Gentiles. (Acts 10)

- Because Peter died, crucified upside down – believing he was not worthy to die like his Lord.

CHAPTER FOUR

So, do we believe that Peter was selected to be the "stone" on which the Christian church was built, but didn't know what he was talking about when he wrote the 1st chapter of 2nd Peter?

Do you think Peter had enough experiences after being a disciple taught by Jesus during Christ's three years of ministry?

Was Peter changed by Christ and the Holy Spirit?

If Peter was chosen by Jesus to lead the flock, should we follow his instruction?

Are the transitions of growth in 2nd Peter, Chapter 1 the same growth Peter had to experience?

Do you think Peter's boldness caused him to proclaim what it takes to be closer to the Lord in his second and last letter to the church?

Are you willing to remove the negative behaviors, idols and problems from your life, like Peter did, so you can make a difference in the world for God?

Peter made many mistakes, but he was chosen by God.

Jesus bluntly pointed out Peter's rash behaviors, but still chose him to lead His sheep.

He was impulsive but became wise through the Holy Spirit.

If we stop and think about it, Peter lived the 12-steps. He could have chosen to continue fishing, but he knew following Jesus was a better life similar to when we choose to leave our old lives behind (step 1). He learned that his Jewish faith was a steppingstone and Christ offered a better world (step 2). He repeatedly developed his faith, watched miracles happening around him, through Christ and even participated in the miracle of walking on water by turning his will and his life over to Jesus (step 3). He continuously struggled with ego but had to inventory his behavior for three days after he denied Christ and was fearful of going to the crucifixion (step 4). I'm sure he was angry with himself, ashamed, and hurt that he did not maintain the love that he proclaimed in front of the 11 other disciples (step 5). In speaking with Jesus after the resurrection he confessed his wrongs to his Lord (step 6). Jesus forgave Peter and the disciples, informing them that the Holy Spirit would come to give them the power to change the world (step 7). The disciples amended their behaviors, waited for Jesus, and humbly accepted the responsibility of continuing Christ's ministry (step 8, 9). When told to stop preaching the news of Christ by the leaders of the church, Peter immediately admitted it would be wrong to listen to men and ignore God (step 10). After Peter was filled with the Holy Spirit, he agreed to take care of Jesus' "sheep" (step 11), was forgiven by Christ and made leader. He then shared the gospel of Jesus Christ and changed the lives of thousands of people in the Jewish faith and eventually Gentiles (step 12).

If Peter led thousands of people to faith, are you willing to follow his instruction through the word of God even though you can't hear him preach at Pentecost?

Peter urges us to "make every effort to respond to God's promises." This is a polite way to say do everything in your strength and receive the blessings of God.

Will you listen and follow Christ?

Will you listen and follow the first disciple and leader of the church assigned by the risen Jesus Christ?

2nd Peter

The most significant location I have found the concept of the 12-steps is in 2 Peter 1:3-13. Those of us in recovery would suggest acquiring a Bible to follow along. I use the New Living Translation Life Recovery Bible.

GROWING IN FAITH

"*3 By His divine power, God has given us everything we need for living a godly life. We have received all of this by coming to know him, the one who called us to himself by means of His marvelous glory and excellence. 4 And because of His glory and excellence, He has given us great and precious promises. These are the promises that enable you to share His divine nature and escape the world's corruption caused by human desires. 5 In view of all this, make every effort to respond to God's promises. Supplement your faith with a generous provision of moral excellence, and moral excellence with knowledge, 6 and knowledge with self-control, and self-control with patient endurance, and patient endurance with godliness, 7 and godliness with brotherly affection, and brotherly affection with love for everyone. 8 The more you grow like this, the more productive and useful you will be in your knowledge of our Lord Jesus Christ. 9 But those who fail to develop in this way are shortsighted or blind, forgetting that they have been cleansed from their old sins. 10 So, dear brothers and sisters, work hard to prove that you really are among those God has called and chosen. Do these things and you will never fall away. 11 Then God will give you a grand entrance into the eternal Kingdom of our Lord and Savior Jesus Christ.*"

PAYING ATTENTION TO SCRIPTURE

"*12 Therefore, I will always remind you about these things—even though you already know them and are standing firm in the truth you have been taught. [13] And it is only right that I should keep on reminding you as long as I live."*

In verse 3, we realize God has provided us with a solution and a way out of every problem we may encounter in our lives. We have no excuse not to live a godly life. We have received these blessings as a result of coming to know God and Jesus. This opportunity occurred because we have responded to God's invitation to know His Son. He extends this invitation because He is full of G.R.A.C.E. (providing us God's Riches At Christ's Expense) and excellent (defined as the quality above standards, extremely good or outstanding). This is the GOD We Serve! Even though we haven't been able to remove ourselves from the predicaments in our lives, He provides us with a way out.

What others may have meant for evil, God uses it for good. If you know Him, you can develop a desire to know Him better! We have been called to have a relationship with Him, REJOICE! Do we have the faith to live the life that Christ has called us to live? Do we serve God to glorify Him or glorify ourselves? Do we walk as we talk? If not, the following verses in Steps 1 through 12 will help us see our call to action.

Step One

We admitted we were powerless over our addictions/hurts/habits/hang-ups - that our lives had become unmanageable.

"⁴And because of His glory and excellence, He has given us great and precious promises. These are the promises that enable you to share His divine nature and escape the world's corruption caused by human desires." 2 Peter 1:4

Because of God's magnificence and inconceivable love for us, He also gives us great and wonderful promises when we surrender to God. What are God's promises? Here are JUST nine of them.

"¹²To all who received him, to those who believed in His name, He gave the right to become the children of God." John 1:12

"¹⁹And this same God who takes care of me will supply all your needs from His glorious riches, which have been given to us in Christ Jesus." Philippians 4:19

"¹¹The LORD will withhold no good thing from those who do what is right." Psalm 84:11

"'¹⁷I will give you back your health and heal your wounds,' says the LORD." Jeremiah 30:17

"³He forgives all my sins and heals all my diseases." Psalms 103:3

"⁸The LORD says, 'I will guide you along the best pathway for your life. I will advise you and watch over you.'" Psalm 32:8

"¹³The temptations in your life are no different from what others experience. And God is faithful. He will not allow the temptation to be more than you can stand. When you are tempted, He will show you a way out so that you can endure." 1 Corinthians 10:13

"² There is more than enough room in my Father's home. If this were not so, would I have told you that I am going to prepare a place for you? ³ When everything is ready, I will come and get you, so that you will always be with me where I am." John 14:2-3

"²⁵And in this fellowship, we enjoy the eternal life He promised us." 1 John 2:25

There are hundreds of promises of wisdom, healing, blessings, peace, eternal life, and solutions to all of our problems. These promises allow us to share in God's divine nature, to be a part of God's family, to be more like Jesus, to be filled and led by God's Holy Spirit.

In **Step 1**, we understand that the pleasures of this world may feel great, but self-indulgence will destroy our lives. We have to ask ourselves some questions...

Which worldly desires control you?

Which idols or people or things do you focus your life on instead of God?

How would you be a better person if you stopped focusing on the addiction?

_____

_____

_____

_____

How would your life be better?

_____

_____

_____

_____

How would you be a better spouse, parent, son, daughter, brother, or sister?

_____

_____

_____

_____

Which fruit of the spirit is limited in your life and what negative behaviors do you need to release to receive them?

_____

_____

_____

What is preventing you from learning and making wise choices?

_____

_____

_____

_____

What are your concerns about letting go of the destructive behavior that would help you to have peace and excitement?

What is preventing you from working with God?

What do you need to change to walk with Him, talk with Him, be with the One who created us to be their best friend?

If you could pick and choose all of the characteristics of your best friend... what would they be?! Would you pick someone like Jesus?

Now imagine if that best friend started hurting themselves, destroying their lives, became obsessed with something that began to damage your friendship, which hurts you. What if someone started hurting your friends? Destroying their lives, marriage, jobs, personality, and thinking? What if the new behavior made them live in a way that continuously crippled them, caused them to self-destruct?

The damage we do to others with our compulsive behaviors is the pain that our loved ones feel when we are in your addiction. If you believe Jesus loves you, don't you think that He feels the same pain? Does God have to look away when you do the corrupt things that He has asked you not to do?

If you are observing your best friend destroying their life, wouldn't you want to intervene? Fix them? Stop them and straighten them out? What if every time you tried to straighten them out, your efforts only impeded their improvement? Could you accept that they need to learn from their mistakes and experiences?

Do we know how to intervene appropriately on a person who's doing damage to their life? If you believe Jesus is all-knowing, do you think He knows the best way to treat your problems? Many families and loved ones try to fix addictive, compulsive behaviors. They have good intentions, but wrong approaches. Some family members are so addicted to fixing their loved ones they become codependent.

As family members, friends, and loved ones, do we realize when we try to fix people, we rob loved ones of:

Growth opportunities;
Healing or Recovery;
Humbly seeking a godly relationship through brokenness
or surrender.

We cannot provide people with eternal life, but only show them and share experiences of our journey with our loving Creator. This is our story, testimony, and our gift from God.

A lady at a codependency meeting was discussing years of attempts to help "straighten out" her husband and her son. After many failed attempts, her insight was, "If I keep fixing the addicts in my life, they never have to learn to rely upon God or recovery." The statement that she didn't make immediately popped in my head (I wonder who that was?) "If I keep fixing the alcoholic or addicts in my life, who am I trying to be?"

The things we want are not always what we need. The attractive, beautiful, desirous possessions of this world are usually not good for us. Sometimes the smallest experience of them will remove us from the path God has purposed for us. We have a choice every day:

- To choose what is right or to determine what is wrong.

- To be for God or against Him.

- To be working on a righteous life or sinful living.

God always provides an out. A friend in recovery repeatedly told me, "God never gives us a test He hasn't given us the answers to." He also stated, "We never fail any of God's tests, we just get to keep taking them over and over and over again until we pass them."

Which worldly desires have corrupted your life? If there is more than one, please write them all.

Have you been unsuccessful in controlling them?

Do thoughts, cravings or obsessions continue to pop up in your mind?

_____

_____

_____

What parts of your life have been negatively impacted by these worldly desires? (Work, school, home, friends, family, emotionally, physically, sexually, spiritually, legally, financially, etc.) Please write one example of each one of these.

_____

_____

_____

_____

_____

_____

_____

_____

_____

_____

_____

_____

_____

Do you want to live a life that is not negatively impacted by decadence?

_____

_____

_____

Step Two

Came to believe that a Power greater than ourselves could restore us to sanity.

"In view of all this, make every effort to respond to God's promises." 2 Peter 1:5a

(Verse 5 encompasses steps 2 through 6 wrapped up in a series of processes and behaviors that God wants us to adopt. Therefore, we will indicate each section of verse 5 as 5a, 5b, 5c, and 5d.)

Here is our reality. I am not going to see a movie that my friends didn't like because we usually have the same interest. I'm not going to go to a restaurant that has poor reviews, because others have told me the food was not good. I check reviews on hotels before I book them. I don't want to work with professionals who have poor reputations, corrupt business practices, are unethical, or provide poor service. When I am going to have surgery, I checked the reviews on the doctor to determine the quality of his work. Whether I am spending my money on something as minor as a meal or a movie or I am making a decision where I'm going to stay, business interactions, or something as serious as surgery, I am going to make sure I am getting the best that I can.

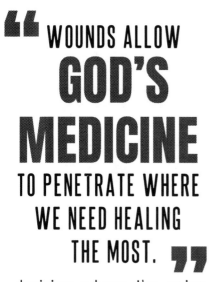

"WOUNDS ALLOW GOD'S MEDICINE TO PENETRATE WHERE WE NEED HEALING THE MOST."

Finding the best service or product also applies to my spiritual walk and my recovery. I want the best counselor for my life struggles. I want to attend churches that fill my spiritual cup and where I can serve and help others. I seek sermons that teach me, reach me and affect my life, so I can, in turn, share my insights with others. In my recovery, I speak with my sponsor at least one time per week. I attend meetings that inspire me to take notes. I listen for words of wisdom I've never heard before and write them down because they are essential to my life and my recovery. I attend at least 3 meetings per week and do as my father did. I asked him one time how often he went to meetings when he had been approximately 20 years sober. He said, "I give (lead) at 2 meetings per week and take (attend) at one. On Wednesday morning, I don't know anything. I am just a person in a meeting who needs help, and I need my cup filled."

My church and my recovery are significant factors in my life. I have gone to churches that have become numb, ritualistic, repetitive, or dutiful. When this happens, I leave the church. I seek churches where the spirit is active, God is working, and healings occur. If I didn't sense God's presence, the filling of the Holy Spirit, or the teachings of Jesus, I would speak to the leadership or go somewhere else.

When I have a problem and am trying to "escape the world's corruption caused by human desires," I go where God is changing lives, and His promises are being fulfilled.

If we ignored God's promises or we informed God that we don't want His gifts or don't want peace and blessings, wouldn't that be insane? We don't reject God outright, instead, we respond to God's offers and promises something like this:

"I would rather have my brief happiness by doing what I want instead of always doing what's right."

"I think I know better than God."

"I know what is right for me!"

"God! You aren't going fast enough."

"I wouldn't have done it that way. I would have done it THIS way."

What we don't see is why He did it the way He did. **HE ALWAYS HAS A BETTER WAY!** We may not like it, but we haven't seen the big picture. He isn't painting a portrait of a moment in time. He is painting an eternity and a universe! A fluid, ever-changing movie that overlaps with billions of other movies all to tell the story of how much He loved you since before you were born. Life is millions of stories of millions of people that belong in His eternal family.

But some chose not to stay in touch. People get angry and never talk to Him again because they can't escape those brief moments in time where resentment locks up their reality and skews their future. So they miss out on the fellowship, the blessings, the promises, the real meaning of true love, and dwell in their small corner of an enormous universe of possibilities. They reject the opportunity to choose eternal life because they become angry with God and His people. They say, "If that is how God is. If that is what His people do, then He must do that too. And I don't want any part of it."

Those moments of temporary insanity become a permanent reality. They cause us to disregard eternity because of our unhealed wounds and distorted perception of life. Our little pit of despair is a minute speck in the universe that becomes a gaping black hole causing us to stop the movie, turn away from God's plan and attempt to right what we think is wrong. Or to respond as a victim. We don't realize the show will go on. God's will is going to be done whether we like it or not, and we will have to rectify our thinking or be left out.

There is a God, and it's not us.

We have to learn to start practicing sober living by realizing He knows better than we do.

We don't have to self-medicate, get high on other people, places, behaviors, or things. All of those desires separate us from those who genuinely love us.

Most of us need to realize our brokenness before we understand that He can help us. We have to come to Him, in pain; hurting, disoriented, and lost. When we are broken, it is easier for God to help us. He will help us if we ask Him. If there is any arrogance within us, and we haven't had enough pain, hurt, or loss, we will still fight His healing. Brokenness is where the spirit shines through the cracks. Wounds allow God's medicine to penetrate where we need healing the most.

We are always hopeful that people find God. Some see Him by the time they're 10 years old, or 18 years old, or 25 years old. Yet others wait until they are 50 or 60 years old before they develop the faith or allow Christ as their Savior. A person may wait 60 or more years before they say a one-minute prayer of total surrender to God, a prayer of Salvation. Christ always accepts us; will we accept Him?

When we have run out of options, when there's nowhere else to go, no one else to turn to, and we have come to the end of our best solutions, then we become willing to accept God's help and seek His direction. Eventually, we realize how much of our lives we have wasted by doing life our way. The blessing is, God will use all of our experiences and testimonies to help someone else develop their faith.

The harsh beauty of recovery is when we have to try everything we can think of to stop our addictive behaviors. When nothing we have attempted works, when our friends and family leave us because of our actions, and we feel completely lost, then God can start to grow and change our lives. But we don't have to wait until we "hit bottom" to change our lives. Sometimes we need the loneliness to realize the significance of our relationship with God. Once we know we need God; He will put people in our lives that can help us.

This is when we decide we want to stop our insane behaviors and learn from others who have overcome the addiction. We will begin to share in the promises that God has laid before us that help us to escape our addiction. When we decide to trust God instead of trusting ourselves, we discover the beauty of God. We see the provision of the world and the purposes of life.

When we believe in ourselves in issues relating to our unhealthy behaviors, we forget it was our decisions that got us into these circumstances. We try to reinvent the wheel and ignore the instructions of God. However, in God's people, we find those who have explored the truths of life and shared them with us. We see these powers more significant than ourselves in God, righteous individuals, fellowships, and writings.

GODLY INDIVIDUALS
(Sponsors and Accountability Partners)

> *"In the same way, you who are younger must accept the authority of the elders. And all of you, dress yourselves in humility as you relate to one another, for "God opposes the proud but gives grace to the humble."* 1 Peter 5:5

Fear and pride have been struggles for humanity and are listed together repeatedly throughout the Scriptures using different words. Accepting authority is an issue for every young person. My father often paraphrased Aristotle by telling me, "If you want to be a good leader, you must be a good follower." I often wanted to take shortcuts and run the show because I thought I knew better. I am sure I'm not alone in this way of thinking.

I remember hearing the story of a man hired to work in upper management of a large national corporation. He was hired and informed that he needed to go to an office on Monday morning where he would receive his uniform. He was trained in the position of a person providing services, inspections, and treatments for customers. He was taught product and company procedures, worked with other service providers, and was dispatched to locations. The next week he learned how to dispatch others, then he learned office management at the corporation of a local office.

Each week he transitioned to the next level of service by working at a regional office, the state office until he had gone through months of training so he could understand how the corporation worked and had an idea of procedures at all levels. He was then placed in his position and had a better understanding of company operations, costs and procedures. Some people will be offended at having to start on the ground floor, but it was necessary to understand in this company.

In Titus 2:1-8, Paul instructs Titus regarding procedures and insights he learned from God and His experience working with Christians. He urges older people to teach younger people, men, women, husbands, wives, behaviors, attitudes, and actions to avoid.

"1 As for you, Titus, promote the kind of living that reflects wholesome teaching. 2 Teach the older men to exercise self-control, to be worthy of respect, and to live wisely. They must have sound faith and be filled with love and patience.

3 Similarly, teach the older women to live in a way that honors God. They must not slander others or be heavy drinkers. Instead, they should teach others what is good. 4 These older women must train the younger women to love their husbands and their children, 5 to live wisely and be pure, to work in their homes to do good, and to be submissive* to their husbands. Then they will not bring shame on the word of God.

*Submission is a difficult word for most people to live by. I have heard many parents and spouses wonder why they are not being respected by their loved ones while they were living in their addictions. At a meeting one time a man introduced himself as an alcoholic, addict, sex addict and rageaholic. He proceeded to complain that his family disrespected him. He couldn't see that stopping these behaviors for a few weeks didn't immediately result in an understanding compliant family. When we are mistreating our family in all of these addictions, why should we think we are deserving of praise. Paulo Coelho quoted, "Respect is for those who deserve it, not for those who demand it." God provides discernment to help us determine if we will follow people who are practicing godly principles or if we are going to submit to destruction and foolishness.

It seems that we can always come up with a better way or better idea. Some people will listen to us, some will take credit for our ideas and others will teach us why our new idea may not be successful. I have been blessed to work with people who have given me opportunities to try different approaches in business and have also been the recipient of their experiences, successes, and failures. God gives us a path to follow by inspiring Paul, who shares the warnings, experiences, and insights he gained from his relationship with God. We see this example in humans who have made mistakes but have been great leaders.

"6 In the same way, encourage the young men to live wisely. 7 And you yourself must be an example to them by doing good works of every kind. Let everything you do reflect the integrity and seriousness of your teaching. 8 Teach the truth so that your teaching can't be criticized. Then those who oppose us will be ashamed and have nothing bad to say about us."

Moses tried to protect a Hebrew worker and killed an Egyptian, but was later chosen by God to set his people free. He didn't know God very well, but many years after murdering the Egyptian, he was called to serve God.

Paul thought he knew God's will and thought he was doing God's work due to his education, heritage, and guidance from his mentors. He killed many people who were believers of Christ until he was struck blind for 3 days. When his physical vision was restored, his heart was also restored as well as a new revelation of Jesus.

King David had everything but then he saw Bathsheba. He broke five commandments (coveting another man's wife, committing adultery, lying, stealing, and murdering) yet he confessed his sin, asked for forgiveness, and was forgiven.

Many people throughout the Scriptures have their insanities exposed. They had mentors, they studied the word of God, they prayed, tried to abide by the commandments, and fellowshipped with others. Even though they made mistakes, they were still God's people who accepted discipline, consequences and received mercy and blessings. This door is open to all of us if we read the Scriptures and see God initiating healing in the lives of his people.

They shared what they learned,

"13 For everyone who calls on the name of the LORD will be saved.

14 But how can they call on Him to save them unless they believe in him? And how can they believe in Him if they have never heard about him? And how can they hear about Him unless someone tells them? 15 And how will anyone go and tell them without being sent? That is why the Scriptures say, 'How beautiful are the feet of messengers who bring good news!'" Romans 10:13-15

Romans 10:13 describes step 2 perfectly. When I first entered recovery, I struggled with the concept of God. It took me seeing others succeeding where I failed, talking about their experiences, finding recovery, finding faith, and surrendering to Him. I was ready to accept because I heard the stories of change and saw people living in assurance.

"42 They devoted themselves to the apostles' teaching and to fellowship, to the breaking of bread and to prayer. 43 Everyone was filled with awe at the many wonders and signs performed by the apostles. 44 All the believers were together and had everything in common. 45 They sold property and possessions to give to anyone who had need. 46 Every day they continued to meet together in the temple courts. They broke bread in their homes and ate together with glad and sincere hearts, 47 praising God and enjoying the favor of all the people. And the Lord added to their number daily those who were being saved." Acts 2:42-47

We all have mentors, teachers, and people who have made an intense impact on our lives. Some of us experience a significant, immediate spiritual infilling of the Holy Spirit, and some of us have a gradual transition. One thing we have learned is that God does whatever He wants to do; however, He wants to do it. He interacts in our lives, and He does it the way He chooses to glorify Him. We learn to give credit where credit is due by praising Him. Seeing His hand in our lives prevents us from thinking we did it ourselves. It prevents us from thinking we have a unique influence over God that causes Him to do whatever "we tell him." It gives us the life experiences and lessons that we need to see His hand in our lives.

They practiced a godly lifestyle,

"13 Therefore, we never stop thanking God that when you received His message from us, you didn't think of our words as mere human ideas. 14 You accepted what we said as the very word of God— which, of course, it is. And this word continues to work in you who believe." 1 Thessalonians 2:13–14

"29 Let no corrupting talk come out of your mouths, but only such as is good for building up, as fits the occasion, that it may give grace to those who hear. 30 And do not grieve the Holy Spirit of God, by whom you were sealed for the day of redemption. 31 Let all bitterness and wrath and anger and clamor and slander be put away from you, along with all malice. 32 Be kind to one another, tenderhearted, forgiving one another, as God in Christ forgave you." Ephesians 4:29-32

We are grateful to be able to practice a recovery lifestyle. Letting go of old behaviors and practicing new behaviors. Healing old wounds and remembering the cure we received because we can see the fading scars instead of the open wounds. We are glad to share how God healed us and his people taught us new ways to live. A saying I heard recently goes, "If you can stay sober one day, you can stay sober a lifetime."

They transitioned from their old way of life into a new way and

"16 All Scripture is inspired by God and is useful to teach us what is true and to make us realize what is wrong in our lives. It corrects us when we are wrong and teaches us to do what is right. 17 God uses it to prepare and equip His people to do every good work."
2 Timothy 3:16-17

They accepted God and His Word

"22 Do not merely listen to the word, and so deceive yourselves. Do what it says." James 1:22

"9 How can a young person stay on the path of purity? By living according to your word." Psalm 119:9

"28 He replied, 'Blessed rather are those who hear the word of God and obey it.'" Luke 11:28

I have been so grateful to be in recovery that was supported by people in 12-step programs, church fellowships, and my own faith. However, discovering 12-step recovery is confirmed by Scripture was something I realized when I returned to the church and deeply examined the word of God. God inspired recovery, it's not just the word of people who are sober. Each day I'm grateful for my recovery, for the peace of mind, and for the second chance I've been given.

GODLY FELLOWSHIPS

"24 Let us think of ways to motivate one another to acts of love and good works. 25 And let us not neglect our meeting together, as some people do, but encourage one another, especially now that the day of His return is drawing near." Hebrews 10:24-25

There may be grumpy old-timers in recovery who are rude or gruff. We can also find these people in churches and church fellowships. However, we can practice living as Jesus did and carrying the message of the disciples, and spreading the good news of all that God has done for us by our testimonies.

CHAPTER FOUR

"¹ Dear brothers and sisters, if another believer is overcome by some sin, you who are godly should gently and humbly help that person back onto the right path. And be careful not to fall into the same temptation yourself." Galatians 6:1

It is our choice to respond to God's promises. Again, we have to consider if it would be insane to avoid the blessings He has for us. People of faith sometimes forget the reason they started or resumed their spiritual walk was because of the kindness of a person filled with God's love who reminded them of the error of their ways and eternal life without God. So, if we would like to have God's blessings, we need to accept God as our personal Savior. This is accomplished in Step 3.

2nd Peter 1:5a	Make every effort to respond to	God's	Promises
Step 2	Came to believe	a power greater than ourselves	could restore us to sanity

Seeing the parallel to step 2 provides me with a greater understanding of God and His promises. It helps me to develop my faith, utilize all the resources that God provides us throughout the Scriptures and stay on track with our healing so we may one day help others find healing.

Which "powers" and spiritual resources are not fully developed in your life? Please explain why.

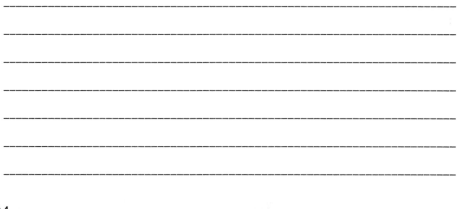

Are you willing to find support in all these areas to help you overcome your issues?

Which one are you not willing to seek out? Why not?

Do you want to keep having the same problems repeatedly, or are you willing to try something new?

Have you ever attended a 12-step meeting?

(Most people in recovery are encouraged to try at least 3 meetings at 2 locations this helps us to find different groups of people that we could relate to better.)

If you have attended and felt uncomfortable in the group, do you realize that other people felt the same way the first time?

_____

_____

_____

_____

Have you ever attended different churches until you found the one that met your needs?

_____

_____

_____

_____

Would you be willing to do the same so you can find healing and learn how to understand yourself?

_____

_____

_____

_____

What are some of the ways your life will be better if you found a trusted fellowship and mentor?

_____

_____

_____

_____

_____

_____

Step Three

Made a decision to turn our will and our lives over to the care of God as we understood Him.

"Supplement your faith." 2 Peter 1:5b

Supplement your faith... Faith requires making a decision, turning our will (what we want to do) and our lives (everything we are) to God as we understand Him (we are building a relationship with Him and it will continue to grow).

In Step 3, we take the step of faith. Faith requires that we make a decision. Faith requires that we turn what we want to do (our will) and everything that we are (our life) to God. Faith is the beginning of understanding God and trusting Him to the degree that we are willing to put our lives in His hands because we believe He is who He says He is and can do what He promises. Faith is the realization that we are not on this earth forever, but we do have an eternity in Heaven with God. Faith is the action we take when we accept Jesus Christ as our personal Savior.

Many churches and people of faith believe Step 3 should be Step 1, and recovery should only be a two-step process: repent and salvation. Unfortunately, most people in 12-step programs take issue with God because of fear, shame, anger, guilt, and depression about their past behaviors. Our unresolved emotions are why Steps 1 & 2 preempt the spirituality of Step 3 by offering reminders of God's love. Step 2 provides an opportunity for people struggling with sinful behaviors to see an opening to God's people who have found proof there is a way out of their damaging lifestyles in Step 1. They have found hope through the promises revealed in their lives, experiences of others in recovery fellowships, and spiritual writings.

So if we know there is a loving God who only wants what's best for us, will we surrender what we want to do and who we are to

Him? Some of us have great fears about surrendering our will and our lives to God. We think He is going to make us do something so contradictory to our beliefs and lives. Our fear of what God will ask of us creates an aversion to trusting Him.

In Jeremiah 29:11-13, God promises that He has plans for us to have a better life to prosper.

"11'For I know the plans I have for you,' says the LORD. 'They are plans for good and not for disaster, to give you a future and a hope. 12In those days, when you pray, I will listen. 13If you look for me wholeheartedly, you will find me.'"

The proof of recovery becomes evident when our lives improve.

When we trust in God;

When we fellowship with other Christians or believers or people of faith and;

When we look at their lives and desire the peace that they have.

Most people in recovery are living a better life and we see proof of the fruit of God.

Sometimes we don't like the cost of a relationship with God. If He is the Creator of the universe, creator of our solar system, the creator of life, creator of time, space, matter, and everything we know, why wouldn't we trust Him? The real question is; <u>why would we trust Him</u>?

Is it because doing what is right doesn't feel as good as our earthly pleasures?

In the action of Step 3 and finding faith in God, we gladly trade our old lives for a new, better existence. Many people only do steps 1-3 and never go further. The "recovery 3 step" usually leads to relapse, switching addictions, or numerous other consequences. As discussed earlier, our resentments, fears, shame, and perceptions of love/sex/intimacy surface as our heads clear.

We briefly lose the obsession to use, but we gain:

- An obsession with retaliation by seeking vengeance on those who we resent because they hurt us in the past.

- Cultivate overwhelming fears of failure, inability to maintain sobriety, losses, and numerous other doubts.

- Practice isolation and shame because we worry about what other people think of us as a result of our old addictive behaviors.

- Nurture reservations of ever being able to have healthy relationships and negative perceptions of self or others due to damaged relationships in the past.

If we want to maintain our recovery, we have to address these issues, which naturally lead us to Steps 4 and 5. It is also the natural path that God laid out for us in the 5th verse.

What is your will?

_____

_____

_____

What is your life?

_____

_____

_____

What are your reservations about turning your will and your life over to God?

_____

_____

_____

CHAPTER FOUR

Do you trust God?

_____

_____

_____

Do you think God has better plans for your life than you do? If you aren't sure, read Jeremiah 29:11-13.

_____

_____

_____

Has God lied to you? OR did He not answer your questions to your liking? List all the situations that you feel He did not answer the way you wanted them answered.

_____

_____

_____

_____

_____

_____

_____

_____

Now, please find someone in recovery or in church ministry that can give you insight into why God may not have answered your questions. List 1-2 people that you believe are wise and would be able to help you with these questions.

_____

_____

_____

What is causing you to not trust in the Lord?

_____

_____

_____

Are there any scriptures that you have found that can answer your questions?

_____

_____

_____

Does God have a greater understanding of the world and life than you have? (Check Isaiah 55:8-9)

_____

_____

_____

It has been said that when Dr. Bob, one of the cofounders of Alcoholics Anonymous ask people if they were ready to turn their will and our lives over the care of God, that he would ask them to "Drop to your knees and accept Jesus as your Savior."

Do you believe that you will be able to stand before God on Judgment Day without having Christ as your advocate? (See John 14:6)

_____

_____

_____

Do you believe you need to turn your will and your life over to God?

_____

_____

_____

Romans 10:9-10 says, if you declare with your mouth, "Jesus is Lord," and believe in your heart that God raised Him from the dead, you will be saved.

"10 For it is with your heart that you believe and are justified, and it is with your mouth that you profess your faith and are saved."

God gives us a choice to believe not just with our minds, but with our hearts. He gives us a choice to proclaim or announce that we believe "Jesus is Lord". Not just quietly mumble it to ourselves, but to share the joy that we have found a solution; we have found God and that we are excited about the opportunity.

"14 But how can they call on him to save them unless they believe in him? And how can they believe in him if they have never heard about him? And how can they hear about him unless someone tells them? 15 And how will anyone go and tell them without being sent? That is why the Scriptures say, "How beautiful are the feet of messengers who bring good news!" Romans 10:14-15

This first sentence of Romans 10:14 identifies the culmination of asking God to save us and believe in Him which aligns with step 3, but can only occur if we have heard of Him in step 2. We only discover God if other people share and profess their experience and relationship with God. We only hear about God if someone was sent to tell us. We are told to share the gospel in Acts 1:8 when Jesus ascended to Heaven and in Matthew 28:16-20 when Jesus gave the disciples the "Great Commission". God wants us to share the good news of second chances, salvation, redemption, and eternal life. People struggling with unhealthy habits and addictions also experience great joy and happiness when they find there is a way out of these addictions as other people share recovery especially when they do their 12th step and carry the message to others.

If you would like to say a prayer accepting Christ as your Savior and trusting in God's word here is a sample prayer you can pray.

Dear Father,

I now believe that Jesus Christ is Your only begotten Son, that He came down to our earth in the flesh and died on the cross to take away all of my sins and the sins of this world. I believe that Jesus Christ then rose from the dead on the third day to give all of us eternal life.

Lord Jesus,

I now confess to You all of the wrong and sinful things that I have ever done in my life. I ask that You please forgive me and wash away all of my sins by the blood that You have personally shed for me on the cross. I am ready to accept You as my personal Lord and Savior. I ask that You come into my life and live with me for all of eternity.

I now believe that I am truly saved and born again. Thank You, Heavenly Father. Thank You, Jesus. Amen

If you want to address your issues relating to the 12-steps, you can say the Third step prayer or something similar.

God, I offer myself to Thee – To build with me and to do with me as Thou wilt. Relieve me of the bondage of self, that I may better do Thy will. Take away my difficulties, that victory over them may bear witness to those I would help of Thy Power, Thy Love, and Thy Way of Life. Amen

Step Four

Made a searching and fearless moral inventory of ourselves.

"...with a generous provision of moral excellence," 2 Peter 1:5c

In Step 4, we do a searching and fearless, MORAL inventory.

A saying repeated in recovery is: "I can't think myself into better behavior, but I can behave myself into better thinking."

God provides us with free will and hopes we are obedient to His word from Genesis to the book of Revelation. Being obedient to a higher authority is how we stay moral. Remembering that we surrender our life and will to Christ (Step 3) is how we stay fearless. Surrounding ourselves with healthier people, a good mentor or sponsor, and living with integrity will make it easier for us to search every aspect of our lives.

When we continue immoral, illegal, and unethical behaviors, we are always living in fear of the authorities finding out, of friends and loved ones leaving us. We do not want to look at every aspect of our lives because we will discover that we are repeating behaviors that continue to cause consequences. Sometimes our greatest fear is what we will find inside of us. In the book, Why Am I Afraid to Tell You Who I Am? By John Powell, we learn:

- We don't want to let people know who we are because they may not like us.

- If we find out who we are, we may not like who we are.

- We are afraid that we are going to find we are terrible people at the core of our being.

Each of these points can be our truth OR cause us to seek a path to a better life. When we read stories in the Scriptures, we learn about other people's mistakes. If we stop and think about it, almost every sin we have committed has been written in the Scriptures.

If we haven't stopped these behaviors, it's because we don't want to look at them. I don't know about you, but I don't know anyone who wants to look at their resentments and resolve them because it helps them feel justified. We don't want to look at how we have hurt others because we feel ashamed. We don't want to explore our fears because there are so many. We don't want to look at how our intimate relationships have been negatively impacted by our behaviors and misconceptions about what love means to us, because we think we know what love is. If we have a difficult time loving others appropriately, it usually is connected to how we love ourselves.

"⁴⁰Instead, let us test and examine our ways. Let us turn back to the LORD." Lamentations 3:40

"²³ For if you listen to the word and don't obey, it is like glancing at your face in a mirror. ²⁴ You see yourself, walk away, and forget what you look like. ²⁵ But if you look carefully into the perfect law that sets you free and if you do what it says and don't forget what you heard, then God will bless you for doing it." James 1: 23-25

What is the perfect law that James is referring to in verse 25? Paul talks about "laws of Christ" in Galatians 6:2. Jesus discussed this perfect law when He spoke to the "expert in religious law" in Luke 10.

The experts summed up the Ten Commandments, which are God's perfect law, into two statements. "You **must** love the Lord your God with all your heart, all your soul, all your strength, and all your mind. And, love your neighbor as yourself."

My question to you is: Can you truly love the Lord your God with all your heart when your heart is corrupted by fear, unforgiveness, shame, self-pity, unhealthy arrogance, and a twisted sense of intimacy?

Look at His instruction in verse 25. *"But if you look underline{carefully into the perfect law..."* How carefully, you ask? Truly evaluate the following questions and explain why.

Do you love God with all your heart, mind, soul, and strength?

Is there something else that you love more than God?

What is the one thing that you keep telling yourself, "God, I will do anything for you, except don't ask me to give up _____ ."

Whatever goes in the blank in the previous sentence, is what you love _more than God_. It is the thing that is preventing you from loving God with every aspect of your being. And, it is preventing you from loving your neighbor as yourself.

Everything you have has been given to you by God. It is for your enjoyment and pleasure, but it was never meant to be more enjoyable or pleasurable than your relationship with God.

Looking carefully into this "perfect law" God promises that it will "set us free" from the bondage of the things that we prioritize over our love for God and God's people (our neighbors). Now I will admit that not all neighbors are lovable, but we have to love them with the love that God would have for them. These attempts at unconditional love and the love that is discussed in 1 Corinthians, chapter 13, is the experience that we have to have that requires "patient endurance" as we continue to progress in reading from the verses in 2 Peter, chapter 1.

James promises that if we *"look carefully into the perfect law"* = are we fully loving God and His people? Are we willing to get rid of the things that we love more than God?

"that sets us free" = if we love God and His people, then we will be set free.

"...and if you do what it says," = don't just read the Scriptures or look at the Scriptures or memorize the Scriptures, but do what the Scriptures say.

"and don't forget what you heard," = don't forget that you gave up (especially whatever you put in the blank) and that your focus needs to be on unconditionally loving God and His people.

"then God will bless you for doing it." = To bless means - to invoke divine care and confer prosperity or happiness upon someone. God will be able to do these things if we are living our life by the perfect law, set free from whatever we idolize, continuing to do what God says, and not forgetting what we heard. We bless God in return, by sharing what God has done for us, by glorifying Him and sharing our testimony. To let people know what we have surrendered to God. In this way, we prove God can be the focus of our lives instead of whatever we idolize or are addicted to.

As a counselor, I have seen many people who live with tremendous guilt, shame, fear, and resentment. It saddens me to think that many people believe this self-examination process is only for alcoholics and addicts. All scriptures are for all people. We are all sinners and all fall short of the glory of God. As indicated above in James 1: 25, we are tempted to carefully examine the perfect law that we receive from God that sets us free. The Scripture promises that if we do what it says and don't forget what we heard that God would bless us for doing it.

In the Scripture from 2 Peter 1:5, regarding how our faith helps develop our moral excellence, we are reminded that we are to seek *"a generous provision of moral excellence."* Step 4 says a *"searching and fearless"* moral inventory. This implies that we should thoroughly examine our behaviors. Nearly a hundred scriptures are urging us to examine our ways, repent, asking God to *"search me,"* acknowledge our weaknesses, test our work, judge ourselves truly, stop condemnation, and be transformed.

Romans 12:2 instructs us to stop the behaviors and habits of this world and let God change us into a new creation.

"Don't copy the behavior and customs of this world, but let God transform you into a new person by changing the way you think. Then you will learn to know God's will (turn over your will) for you, which is good and pleasing and perfect."

The customs and behaviors of this world damaged our lives (Step 1). Believing that God can transform us into a new person and change the way we think (trusting that God will help us think and understand more clearly is step 2) and learning God's will for us makes our life "good and pleasing and perfect" is the blessing of step 3. We can have the strength and faith to face our fears, resentments, and shame.

If we do explore these negative aspects of our lives, we soon discover that we don't want to live like this anymore. We will cautiously and optimistically admit them to God, ourselves, and others, which leads us to Step 5.

(Note: There is a worksheet that you can find on the Internet that helps identify resentments, fears, and harm we have perpetrated on others. Writing this step, speaking with others, and coming to a healthy conclusion requires interactions with those who have completed this step. Being involved with a 12-step support group, people who have over a year of sobriety and have worked all 12-steps are the best resources to find healing. Please have a support network in place before you do steps 4 and 5.)

Why do you think God tells us to examine **ALL** of our ways?

Look at Proverbs 5:21, *"For the LORD sees clearly what a man does, examining **every** path he takes."*

Lamentations 3:40 says, *"Instead, let us test and examine our ways. Let us turn back to the Lord."*

Is God only asking us to examine the easy stuff? Or does he want you to examine everything?

If you are still concerned, read Psalm 139 and realize that God knew you before you were born, knew every day of your life, and everything about you. We cannot confess, what we do not examine and share. God wants us to confess to others and to Him. (1 John 1:9, James 5:16). If you are having a difficult time doing this, go back to Step 3 and determine if you trust God to help you strip away everything. We must trust him so he can cleanse us. Please write a prayer surrendering all your fears, resentments and shame in the space below.

Step Five

**Admitted to God, to ourselves, and to another human being
the exact nature of our wrongs.**

"...moral excellence with knowledge" 2 Peter 1:5d

Upon the conclusion of writing this inventory, we proceed to share the writing in Step 5. Sharing this inventory helps us understand who we are, why we do what we do, and who we could be if we stop the behaviors by allowing God to take control in our lives.

We had a difficult time looking at our lack of morals because we were just looking out for our well-being. However, when we contemplate that we need to talk to someone else about our decline in ethical behaviors, our anxiety returns. The fear of rejection, judgment, and concern about revealing our weaknesses to others reminds us of how people in our past have used our "secrets" against us. What we fail to recall is that the person we are usually sharing our inventory with has already shared their inventory with someone else in recovery. We have entered into a fellowship of people who understand the need to be safe and appropriate with the information of past indiscretions. People in recovery understand how the healing process can be stopped by someone violating that trust.

If we decide to trust God and our sponsor, we will realize that we are entering into a spiritual fellowship of people who have worked with God to find their recovery. People who have found healing are happy to aid others to find healing.

"Confess your sins to each other and pray for each other so that you may be healed. The earnest prayer of a righteous person has great power and produces wonderful results." James 5:16

In James 5: 16, our sins wound us. The healing process begins when we share our sins and we pray for each other. Another aspect of step 5 is realizing that this practice is spiritual behavior. God tells us to confess to one another and if we betray one another, we betray God. The inventory process urges us to invite God, ourselves, and another human being to this confession and healing process.

"But if we confess our sins to Him, He is faithful and just to forgive us our sins and to cleanse us from all wickedness." 1 John 1: 9

In 1 John 1:9, we learn that by confessing to another person, we are also confessing to God. God promises that He is faithful, a just God that forgives and cleanses us of our negative behaviors. God will forgive if only we will ask. We have to take what has been concealed in the darkness and expose it to the light.

"For once you were full of darkness, but now you have light from the Lord. So live as people of light!" Ephesians 5:8

Ephesians 5:8 helps us realize that God and others know that we have all walked in darkness, but now we have the healing, redeeming light of God to help us stay focused on being godly people. However, it only happens if we are willing to expose it and be honest.

Throughout all of the scriptures, God has asked people to stop their evil ways, repent, confess, admit, along with numerous other words that indicate the need to heal. When we complete Step 5 by sharing it with God and one other person, we also share it with ourselves. When we are in therapy or speaking with others about our problems or someone asks us a question that makes us think, sometimes we hear ourselves say something we have never heard before. I heard an amazing statement at a 12-step meeting:

My ears need to hear
my mouth say
what my heart knows.

Confession without change is a lie. When we confess our anger and resentments, how do we feel inside?

If we hold onto those resentments, how will our lives get better or worse?

Should we forgive others even though they don't ask?

Does God want us to resent or forgive? Why?

When we live in fear are we living a full life or half of our lives?

_____

_____

_____

_____

If you think you need to hold onto your fear, think about what 2 Timothy 1:7 (NLT) says, *"For God has not given us a spirit of fear and timidity, but of power, love, and self-discipline."*

How much different would your life be if you could let go of all of your fears?

_____

_____

_____

_____

_____

If the spirit of fear doesn't come from God, where does it come from?

_____

_____

_____

_____

Is it possible to overcome the things we are ashamed of having done in our past?

_____

_____

_____

_____

Steps Six & Seven

***

Step 6 - Were entirely ready to have God remove all these defects of character.

Step 7 - Humbly asked Him to remove our shortcomings.

"...and knowledge with self-control," 2 Peter 1:6a

As we gain KNOWLEDGE of our moral shortcomings, we can:

"Escape (from) the world's corruption caused by human desires". **2 Peter 1:4.**

(Step 1 - by admitting we had a problem that we couldn't control, a problem that damaged our lives and caused us to rely more on unhealthy behaviors and pain than healthy living and peace.)

Develop insight to help us obtain the confidence to *"make every effort to respond to God's promises".*

(Step 2 - by coming to believe/respond to God's promises to help us overcome negative behaviors)

Develop assurance to help us decide to "supplement our faith".

(Step 3 - by enhancing or magnifying our belief as a result of total trust in God when we turn who we are and all of our decisions to God.)

Develop wisdom to differentiate right from wrong. We prepare to let go of harmful practices *"with a generous provision of moral excellence."*

(Step 4 helped us to search every aspect of our lives fearlessly. Step 5 enabled us to demonstrate this moral excellence by acknowledging our part in fear, resentments, the harm we have done to others, and false intimacy. Both steps 4 & 5 helped us to surrender our entire being. We confess to one person who has experienced the humbling, healing process. We become aware of factors that corrupted our morals, thoughts, and lives. We conclude by acknowledging to God who can heal us and forgive us of all our past indiscretions. We become willing to be transformed.)

In Step 6, we become willing to remove these defects of character that we have found in our addictive lifestyle. We ask God to help us stop the justification we developed while living in that lifestyle. Because of our lack of faith, our trust in our unhealthy behaviors, or chemicals, _we stopped trusting God_. We had to decide to let go of unhealthy beliefs we discovered in our inventory. Very few people, (even those who know they have defects of character) rarely stop any behaviors or habits, no matter how destructive. When we know we have defects, we don't know how to stop them. Surrender is one of the main reasons for this book; to understand that living under our shame, guilt, and idolizing addictive behaviors prevents us from being who God created us to be. God has instructed us to become aware and let Him reveal a new and better life. This only becomes available to us when we let go of the old way of living and seek a new life. This whole process reminds me of who Jesus was:

The Way. The path that we are following.

The Truth. The revelation, confession, and change.

The Life. We become a new creation because of Jesus Christ's revelation.

Many people make the mistake of problem-based recovery/ spirituality versus solution-based recovery/spirituality. What I mean by this is that we are trying to avoid negative behaviors instead of practicing positive behaviors. We are struggling to stop doing what we want versus doing what we need. Despite all we have learned about ourselves, we continue to want to "sit on the fence." Sitting on the fence prevents us from totally letting go of our old life in the hope we can also have our new better life (just in case it gets too boring). We know the immediate gratification we get from our negative behaviors; however, we rarely consider their long-term consequences. If we stay focused on the solution of practicing self-control by practicing or improving our assets instead of avoiding defects, we make more progress. These practices give us hope instead of fear.

What old defects of character are you afraid to release?

Is there an ideal behavior that you could be practicing that would be better?

Have you been unsuccessful in releasing this behavior in the past?

Do you think God wants you to hang on to this defective behavior?

Are you willing to let it go now?

In Step 7, we pray for God to remove these defects, and **we** replace them with faith, forgiveness, humility, and love. These replacements are attributes we have learned in recovery or our Christian walk. We continuously practice this SELF-CONTROL and begin the process of repairing the damage. We practice this self-control not by stopping behaviors that we couldn't control but by practicing new actions we can control. This revelation helps us understand that: *when we can't stop our unhealthy behaviors, we start practicing healthy behaviors.*

God points out the negative attributes of a sinful life without Him throughout the scriptures. If 2 Peter 1:6 was focused on negatives, it would urge us to understand that, "ignorance is replaced with self-destruction and self-destruction with demanding impatience and demanding impatience transitions to godlessness." The actual Scripture is worded as: "knowledge with self-control, and self-control with patient endurance, and patient endurance with godliness". This passage of 2nd Peter reveals the concept of overriding the negative with the positive by only focusing on the positive. In 2 Peter 1:6, we transform when we grow in Christ by understanding who we are, why we do things, stopping bad behaviors, asking God to help us practice righteous living, and enduring the growth process with patience.

In **Steps 6 and 7**, we reach the midpoint of the 12-steps. We begin to see the benefit of trading out detrimental defects of character for positive assets. If we honestly review what we have done so far in the 12-steps, we will see that we have been trading out defects for assets since Step 1 and will continue to do so through to step 12. We can see in Step 1, where we traded the decadent worldly behaviors for honesty and righteous living. In Step 2, we see that we couldn't do it ourselves, so we sought help. We repeatedly made the same mistakes; however, recovery taught us that we needed to start relying upon God and others so that we could stop our mistakes. In Step 3, we traded out our "do it yourself" attitudes for surrendering our will and life to God. In step 4, we traded out our avoidance of looking at our past indiscretions by doing a "searching and fearless moral inventory." In step 5, we realize that keeping our secrets to ourselves would prevent us from the honest assessment and the healing of sharing these problematic behaviors with man and God. We continue to see this all the way through to Steps 6 and 7 where we become willing to let go of behaviors that didn't work well for us and trade them for a spiritual walk of positive actions.

As we continuously practice these positive actions, we replace our:

- fear with faith

- resentments with forgiveness

- arrogance with humility

- criticism with gratitude

- hate with love

I am always amazed at how many people are hesitant to give up their defects of character. I believe that we are holding onto these defects because we don't know how we would live our lives without them. Especially since they are unhealthy for those around us and continue to do damage to our lives.

What unhealthy behaviors are you afraid to release from your life?

_____

_____

_____

Are you willing to give up:

Dishonesty? _____

Selfishness? _____

Low Self-esteem and Humiliation? _____

Arrogance? _____

What other negative coping skills will you give up and replace to learn positive coping skills?

_____

_____

_____

_____

_____

If you haven't been able to stop them on your own, do you believe God can help you release them?

_____

_____

_____

How will your life be better if you give up the negative for the positive?

_____

_____

_____

Do you see how exploring your history teaches you who you are and why you react in certain ways can transition to self-control? This is why the growth and insight we gain in Steps 4-7 help us to practice self-control but God also reminds us to be resolute and persistent with ourselves as God is towards us.

CHAPTER FOUR

In my recovery, I have been so grateful for the transition of knowing myself better and being renovated through healthy practices and recovery. This is why I love the Scripture in 2 Peter 1:6 *"knowledge with self-control, and self-control with patient endurance, and patient endurance with godliness."*

It eventually becomes clear that the hurt we have imposed upon others needs to be resolved. Changing our behavior leads us to **Steps 8 through 10** and the next part of verse 6.

In recovery, we say 7th step prayer something like this: *My Creator, I am now willing that you should have all of me, good and bad. I pray that you now remove from me every single defect of character which stands in the way of my usefulness to you and my fellows. Grant me strength, as I go out from here, to do your bidding. Amen*

Please pray this prayer or write one below before you move on to the next chapter.

Steps Eight, Nine, & Ten

Step 8 - Made a list of all persons we had harmed, and became willing to make amends to them all.

Step 9 - Made direct amends to such people wherever possible, except when to do so would injure them or others.

Step 10 - Continued to take personal inventory and when we were wrong promptly admitted it.

"...self-control with patient endurance," 2 Peter 1:6b

A friend who reviewed this writing commented, "Self-control with patient endurance from verse 6, feels forced because those 5 words do not indicate a concept of making amends." I beg to differ. Let's look at a few definitions from Merriam-Webster's dictionary that encompass this process that we are practicing.

Definition of apologize - *to express regret for something done or said: to make an apology. He apologized for his mistake.*

Definition of make amends - *to do something to correct a mistake that one has made or a bad situation that one has caused. She tried to make amends by apologizing to him.*

Definition of self-control - *restraint exercised over one's impulses, emotions, or desires.*

Okay, so here is my point. Practicing restraint is an ongoing process. Control over our impulses, emotions, or desires is a lifetime process. When we let go of one type of desire, we may experience new desires, impulses, or feelings that we have to endure patiently throughout our lives.

Definition of patient - *remaining steadfast despite opposition, difficulty, or adversity.*

How often do we practice patience in our life?

Do we practice patience one time and become perfect at it? Do we ever have to practice patience again for the same situation?

Throwing in the definition of impatient (dictionary.com): *restless in desire or expectation; eagerly desirous.*

Most of us practice patience every day all day long.

Definition of endurance - *the ability to sustain a prolonged stressful effort or activity*

We **PATIENTLY ENDURE** the process of practicing self-control by being aware of our impulses, emotions, or desires that have become habits and automatic responses to situations. God has removed those weaknesses from us. Now, we have to find replacement behaviors and develop new coping skills. By consciously focusing on the fact that we are not going to resort to our old conduct and start practicing new spiritual recovery-related actions, we will be able to amend past wrongs.

We **PATIENTLY ENDURE** implementing new positive behaviors instead of resorting back to our old coping skills.

We **PATIENTLY ENDURE** the old desire of *just apologizing* by saying, "I'm sorry, I promise not to do it again" with *amending our behaviors* by saying, "I apologize for doing that, AND I am making every effort never to do that again. I'm sorry I did it to you, can you forgive me?" In these steps, we learn to take responsibility for our behaviors and stop making excuses for them. We have been changed in Steps 6 and 7 and we quit blaming others because our behaviors are our responsibility. Ultimately, we acknowledge, "What I did was wrong and I am here striving to live differently."

If anyone thinks this does not require self-control **with** patient endurance, you probably have not worked the 12-steps.

Once we move to **step 8**, the apprehension we feel about amending our past wrongdoings is usually one of the greatest obstacles to overcome. I have met and worked with many people who are stuck at step 6 or 7 because they fear repercussions of making amends, rejection, anger, retaliation, or revenge.

Writing a list of people we have harmed, thinking about the negative things that we brought to their lives by our sinful behaviors, and amending our conduct is a fear that many people hold on to for their entire lives. I have seen people who will not attempt to stop using drugs and alcohol, overeating, binging and purging, gambling, etc. People won't seek therapy or stop acting out sexually because "I don't want to make a promise I can't keep." We have to remember we can't make that promise of our own fruition. It takes support from God and His people. Writing the list, preparing a script isn't necessarily the hard part (Step 8), the difficult part is: are we going to be able to keep our promise (Steps 6 and 7)?

Are we going to be able to fulfill our act of contrition and stop the behavior that we have amended to those we offended?

In Step 9, we think about what we are going to say to the people we have done wrong. We discuss our approach with our sponsor. We meet with the easiest people first. We find the right place, the right time, and reach out to them. We patiently endure and seek these people, which we may not be able to find for months or even years. The amazing thing about God is that when it is time to make amends, the right place and the right time will present themselves. We may not have been able to find or see this person for years, then suddenly they will reappear in our lives.

We persist in addressing our past and reconciling relationships as it provides healing to us and healing to others. Some people may not accept our attempt at reconciliation, but we are the ones who need to start the healing process. Forgiveness will lay in the hands of the people we have asked.

The next verse after the end of the Lord's prayer, Matthew 6:14-15, quotes Jesus as saying, *"If you forgive those who sin against you, your heavenly Father will forgive you. But if you refuse to forgive others, your Father will not forgive your sins."*

A college who reviewed this book stated that the Scripture in Matthew 6:14-15 (quoted above) is "not my theology" as it indicates a vengeful God and causes people to feel guilty. It seems today that when people select a "God of their own understanding" that they choose all the nice, pretty ideas from spirituality without looking at the responsibility and consequences of behaviors. God is a God of grace and mercy, yet he does hold us to a standard. If we say that Jesus didn't really

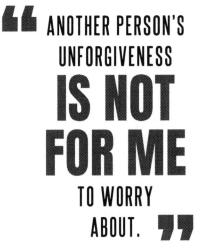

ANOTHER PERSON'S UNFORGIVENESS IS NOT FOR ME TO WORRY ABOUT.

mean what he said in Matthew 6:14-15, does that mean that the Golden Rule does not apply either? Does that mean that we can do onto others without expecting any consequences? Does that mean God is not going to give people consequences for their behaviors like he did with King David, Paul, and everyone else in the Bible? Does this mean that if we are offended by any words in the Scriptures that we can cross them out and disregard them? If that's the case, we would have to pass the scriptures in the Bible around to everyone and allow them to cross out what they did not believe was true, or whatever made them feel guilty or what they didn't like. Eventually, if the last 3 words left in the Bible were that, "God is love," I'm sure someone would be angry and offended enough about circumstances in their life that they would probably cross that out too. So did Jesus make that statement because God is spiteful? Is Jesus lying? Is he trying to intimidate us into good behaviors? Do God or Jesus discuss parables in Proverbs and not mean them? Is God loving by telling us the truth whether we like it or not or is He codependent by telling us only what we want to hear?

You already know the answer to those questions. If Jesus did not maintain God's standards, He would not be a just God. God has offered peace to us; we need to offer peace to others.

Now, back to the discussion on forgiving/not forgiving those who sin against us and God forgiving/not forgiving us. I am thinking, "Whoa!" I do not want to use my power of forgiveness or lack of forgiveness for God to pull out the Golden Rule on me. "Do unto others as you would have them do unto you". Jesus tells the parable of the unmerciful servant in Matthew 18:21-35. The man who was forgiven of much and received mercy from the king did not forgive someone who owed him little and had consequences from the king. That parable starts with the words, "The Kingdom of Heaven is like...".

I will release others from the bondage of my resentments borne of my unforgiveness. I will release the power of my unforgiveness, so I can have peace. So we can have peace. They may not be ready to forgive me, but I have opened the door. Just like I have to find forgiveness in my heart through working with God, they will have to make the same decision and may need to ask God to give them the insight, strength, or peace to forgive me.

Another person's unforgiveness is not for me to worry about. I do need to be genuine, compassionate, and sincere in my amends process. I need to let God work in me and work in the other person. If they do not forgive me and they tell me they will never forgive me, the bitterness they have harbored will be on their mind. They may forgive me in private or they may one day approach me and tell me that my act of asking for forgiveness opened the door to a life in recovery, a faith life, and healed many of their damaged relationships.

The unforgiveness of others will also be on my mind to help me remember the damage my unhealthy habits have inflicted on other people's lives, encouraging me to continue working on my recovery so I never do it again to anyone else. It helps me to constantly seek God so I can be a better person each day. Some people might go in the other direction when they are not forgiven by becoming depressed, angry, and wounded.

Recovery teaches us not to dwell on self-pity, low self-esteem, and ego. On page 88 in the Alcoholics Anonymous big book, it states, "but we must be careful not to drift into worry, remorse or morbid reflection, for that would diminish our usefulness to others". This type of self-pity and behavior draws attention back to me instead of glorifying God for the forgiveness process that He has provided. God had to wait for us to change our lives and even come to this point of seeking forgiveness. As we consider that now is our time to start this process, God will inspire those we interact with to start their own healing process. God will never give us more than we can handle (1 Corinthians 10:13).

I don't think we realize the damage we have done in our faith and our twisted perception of spirituality. We forget how we have used spiritual principles and spiritual words to justify our bad habits and unhealthy behaviors. We don't seek God, we just think we know what He would do even though we don't know Him. I have had discussions with many people who deflect an idea or Scripture that is out of context to manipulate a situation. If we have done any of the aforementioned behaviors, we may need to make amends to God. (I said "May" to be polite.) We all sin and most of us sin multiple times daily. And if you think you are without sin and have nothing to make amends for, God has some Scriptures for you.

The best way we can make amends to God is by:

- Living the life He asked us to live (discovered in the Scriptures)

- Being who He created us to be (revealed in our relationship with Him)

- Glorifying Him instead of ourselves (revealed in the humility and life of Christ; as He sought to do His Father's work)

We ensure that we are resolving issues with people "we have harmed" to release the bondage of shame that has limited our interactions with others and has caused others to be wary of "people like us". In the recovery process and the transformation that Peter has asked us to live in these verses, we can glorify God, demonstrate the viability of the Scriptures, and show that God can change us to a new man or woman. When reminded of our past indiscretions, we can agree that we were that way at one time but we are doing everything we can to be our best selves at this time. Step 10 is the proof of inventorying our past behaviors that may arise again, looking at our defects of character and "when wrong, promptly admitting it." This lets people know we are still a work in progress. This lets us know that when we make mistakes, we can practice new and better behaviors to resolve them.

We make the amends to restore relationships because we know we have done wrong. After exploring our inventory and our defects of character we know that many of the conflicts we have had in the past were because of our issues. The saying, "time heals all wounds" does not bear true in many situations. Wounds that are not healed, will fester and our woundedness will be transmitted to others. Think about trying to help a wounded animal. If you get your hand near the object of their pain or wounds they will snarl and snap at you. This is the same way we are if we have unresolved issues in our lives.

Hurting people, hurt people.

Wounded people, wound people.

However, **Healing people, heal people.**

In Step 10, we continue PATIENTLY to ENDURE the recovery process daily. We practice these principles of inventorying our behavior, stopping negative behavior, seeking better behaviors, and correcting our mistakes. We begin to think about people we had harmed daily and immediately make amends to them in our daily lives.

The reason **patient endurance** fits so well for Steps 8, 9 & 10 is not for the fact that it takes 30 to 60 minutes to write the list in Step 8 but rather that it may take days, weeks, months, or even years of patience (and anticipation) to find the people that are owed resolutions for our past indiscretions. It also takes practice to implement new behaviors.

Some of us may avoid making amends for:

- Fear of looking foolish.

- Concerns about the anger of others.

- Experiencing the fear that opening up old wounds will create problems instead of blessings.

On some occasions, we may believe the person we are trying to make amends to owes us an apology for their behaviors. Even if that is the case, we need to resolve **our** issues so we can continue to live in peace. If we do not address our past indiscretions, we will not be able to resolve our present errors and progress to the next steps or progress as Peter has outlined in this chapter.

When we make amends to someone, we should not expect them to think about any amends or apologies they may owe us. Sayings I have heard in recovery reveal that "expectations are planned resentments" or "expectations are planned failures". Hardly anything goes the way I "expect" them to go so I should do what God asks me to do and pray that His will be done. Remember, you have been living a spiritual life and/or working the 12-steps, inventoried your behavior, asked God to change you, and are now cleaning up the wreckage of your past. People may not believe you and think you are only trying to manipulate them. It's our responsibility to work on our recovery and their responsibility to work on their personal growth.

Whether people forgive us or not, the responsibility is theirs. In Steps 4 and 5, we privately forgave anybody who trespassed against us, but in steps 8, 9, and 10, we are to seek forgiveness for any harm or damage we've done to others. This is one of those promises that Peter spoke of in verse 4, "the promises that enable you to share His divine nature and escape the world's corruption caused by human desires." I will continue to identify more promises throughout this book.

I have patiently endured growing out of the immaturity of what I thought the world should be like and learned that the plan God has for me is better than anything I can imagine. I am grateful and willing to explore where my unhealthy behaviors came from, release my defects of character and heal damaged relationships. Mending relationships is the blessing of the "amends steps". Our deliberate purpose is to resolve our past indiscretions no matter the cost, trials, or suffering we must endure. We do not enter this step with cowardice or revenge, but with self-restraint and a desire to resolve these past destructive behaviors.

If you have been working with a sponsor as you're going through each one of these chapters, then you are ready to do this step. If you think you need to make amends to someone at this very moment without contemplating where the behavior came from, without asking God to remove your defects of character because you want the immediate gratification of resolutions to relationships, _you are working on your schedule, not God's timing_. Second Peter has laid out this transformation process for a reason. The reason was: Peter received a revelation from God. Living In our "participation award", "immediate gratification", "microwave world" we think we can bypass what God asks us to patiently endure. In recovery, we learn to "trust the process". Self-medicating and treating ourselves without seeking help from others, or God is egotistical, arrogant, and fear-filled. You do not put gauze and tape on a wound. You rinse it, disinfect it, and then apply the bandage. Applying the gauze, then applying the antiseptic followed by rinsing it will cause your wounds to fester and your problems to be intensified.

Would you like to restore damaged relationships?

Who are the people that need to be on your list of amends and what amends do you need to make to each of them?

Would you like to restore damaged relationships?

Does God say to patiently endure for only a week or month?

How will your life improve if you clean up the damage that you did to relationships?

_____

_____

_____

_____

What negative feelings dominate this amends process? For each negative feeling, explain your reservation.

_____

_____

_____

_____

_____

_____

_____

What are the positive feelings that you can perceive by doing the amends process?

_____

_____

_____

_____

_____

_____

_____

We may not think there will be anything positive, but who are the ultimate beneficiaries of amending and healing past relationships?

If you can stop negative patterns of your past, can you start new and better patterns each day?

Step 10 makes a point that we aren't going to be perfect but we can get better.

Continued to take personal inventory and **when we were wrong** promptly admitted it.

Here is the patient endurance. Just like we have to be aware of our behaviors when we become Christians and start practicing worldly behaviors and beliefs, we have to patiently endure changes in our lives to be more Christ-like. As we become more like Christ, we are led to step 11 and what is revealed in 2 Peter 1:6: "patient endurance with godliness".

Step Eleven

Step 11 - Sought through prayer and meditation to improve our conscious contact with God as we understood Him, praying only for knowledge of His will for us and the power to carry that out.

"...and patient endurance with godliness,..." 2 Peter 1:6c

Patiently enduring the growth process, cleaning up our wreckage, and repairing relationships provides us with an opportunity that leads us to godliness (Step 11). Praying and meditating also require patient endurance. Think about how many times we have prayed, opened our eyes, and immediately hoped our "wish had been granted." My God seems to be a God of last-minute answers. I receive insights on teachings, problems, and solutions shortly before resolutions are required. Waiting on God has taught me (most of the time) to trust that God will do what He said he's going to do. Some prayers I have prayed for days, weeks, months, and years but they are always answered.

Even meditation requires patient endurance. Sometimes we can meditate on God's word and not receive any significant answer only to find that solutions come through living and experiencing life. There have been times where we can quietly meditate for substantial periods and others where our mind is racing, and we can't hear God.

Side note: When I have a difficult time maintaining stability and calm during meditation, I keep a pen and notepad near me. If racing thoughts persist, I write them down so I can let them go and listen to God. Writing helps me to help me focus and document insights that come from meditation or to ensure that I take care of a persistent thought or responsibility that needs resolution when I finish my meditation.

We don't always get what we pray for, and meditation doesn't always go as planned, but in all things, we can learn. We seek out His plans for us to be better people. We revere and respect His wishes. Prayer is one of the most significant ways that we can respect God. We glorify Him, we thank Him, we praise Him, and hopefully, we will listen to Him. Listening to Him, knowing and seeking His answers from the Scriptures, being mindful of His promptings, and listening to those He has blessed with spiritual insights and wisdom are ways that we can meditate on His word.

The joy we receive from prayer and meditation encourages us to help others. We want to share the wonderful experiences we have had and reveal how we endured through difficult times with His strength and reassurance. Sharing this experience and our new desire to help others is what leads us to Step 12.

*How much time are you spending per day **speaking** to the Creator of the universe?*

----

*How much time are you spending per day **listening** to the Creator of the universe?*

Are you obeying Him?

If you are speaking to Him, but not hearing Him, attend church, a Bible study, or a recovery meeting and start practicing what you hear others incorporating into their lives. God will speak to you through a still small voice, other people, Scriptures, sermons, the Bible, recovery literature, lost opportunities, and new opportunities.

What are some of the times and words you have received from God that blessed your life?

What was the last thing He told you to do that you have **not** *done yet?*

What have you allowed to get in the way of doing what God asked you to do? Sometimes our lives will be on hold until we obey our last instructions.

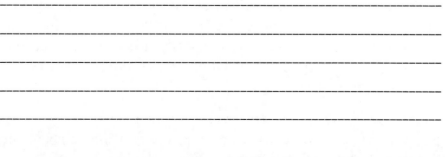

Step Twelve

Step 12 - Having had a spiritual awakening as the result of these steps, we tried to carry this message to others and to practice these principles in all our affairs.

"...and godliness with brotherly affection, and brotherly affection with love for everyone." 2 Peter 1:7

Webster's Dictionary defines godliness as "believing in God and in the importance of living a moral life."

This verse is so loaded with opportunities to serve God and His people. It provides us with compassion and understanding for the struggles of others. By this time in our recovery fellowships, we have seen demonstrations of support, strength, service, wisdom, experience, hope, faith, love, and many other ways to exhibit affection. As we continue to practice speaking to God and listening to God, we are prompted to help others who have struggled with problems similar to ours. We reach out to our brothers and sisters, we become more available to them as sponsors/mentors, and share the principles of recovery (Step 12) to help them live the new lives that we've been given. Serving is a demonstration of God's love. Jesus demonstrated the servant attitude by healing, helping, teaching, practicing humility, and serving. Attending to the needs of others exemplifies the healing and help that many of the Saints of faith have provided to the struggling, the less fortunate, or people in need. As we practice these behaviors with people in recovery, we begin to find subtle ways to incorporate them in every area of our lives and interact with everyone in a healthy way. We begin to share the love that was given to us when we were down and out and provide comfort to others.

In recovery, we learn that we have to give it away to keep our sobriety. In our Christian walk, we continue to gain new experiences and insight into the lives of our brothers and sisters. We learn new ways to serve from God.

Have you ever been prompted to do something such as pray for someone? I was at a hospital one day visiting some friends. I noticed a family who appeared stressed while waiting for news of the medical condition of their loved one. God told me to pray for them. I went where they were seated and asked if I could pray for them. The words came, I prayed, they cried and one of the family members said, "Thank you, we didn't know what to do, we were praying for an answer and that was the answer to our prayer."

Our recovery experience is just like our Christian walk. When we receive the good news of the gospel of Jesus Christ, we want to share it with others. When we are finally able to stop a destructive habit through the power of God, we want share that in meetings. Sometimes we are bothered by the boldness that we see with people who will walk up to us in a parking lot and ask us, "If you died today, do you know where you would end up?" The reason some Christians have such boldness is because they are glad to share the message of Jesus Christ. They want others to experience the freedom of redemption from sin in their lives and hope to encourage others to choose to live in eternity with God. The reason we become bold in our recovery is that we were thrilled to share the good news of what Jesus Christ has given us. We are grateful that God removes addiction from our lives and enthusiastically share how we are developing our faith and a sober mind; both of which are gifts from God. Living like this brings joy back into this world and supreme happiness with God in the next.

Are you ready to share what God has given you?

Are you ready to carry the message to new people coming into church and recovery?

_____

_____

_____

_____

Are you ready to lead meetings, Bible studies, recovery book studies based on what you have learned about yourself?

_____

_____

_____

_____

Are you ready to share what you have learned about God?

_____

_____

_____

_____

Are you ready to share Your faith and your recovery?

_____

_____

_____

_____

It does not take a Masters' degree in divinity or counseling to share your faith or your recovery. It only requires you to share your experience, strength, and hope. Will you share your faith and recovery the next time you are prompted by God?

Romans 10:14-15 says "*14 How, then, can they call on the one they have not believed in? And how can they believe in the one of whom they have not heard? And how can they hear without someone preaching to them? 15 And how can anyone preach unless they are sent?*" As it is written: "How beautiful are the feet of those who bring good news!"

If you have found recovery, do you think others would like to know about it too?

_____

_____

_____

_____

Would you like someone to help you find recovery and healing?

_____

_____

_____

_____

Are you willing to share recovery with others just as I am now sharing it with you?

_____

_____

_____

_____

CONTINUING OUR WALK

The Promise of Growth

Forgetting to Remember

"Works" to Remember Faith

Obedience Provides a Blessing

How Long Do We Have to

Do This?

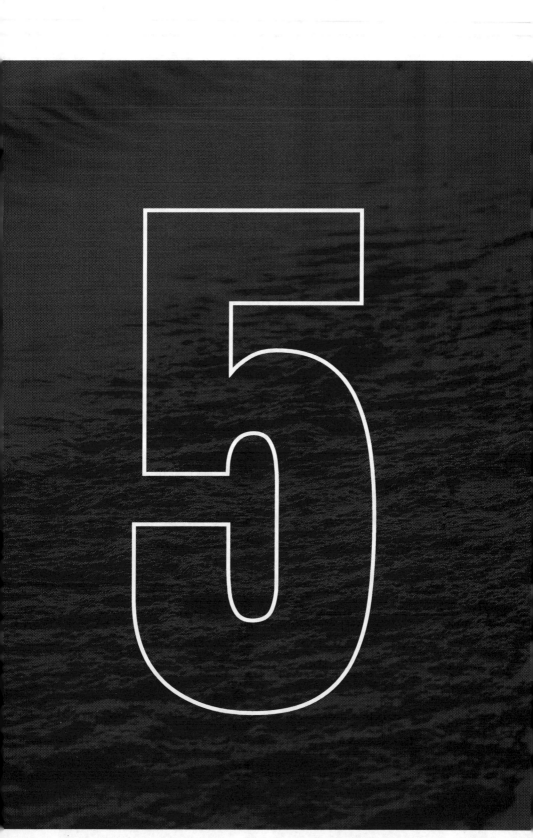

chapter four
CONTINUING OUR WALK

The Promise of Growth

The astonishing thing about this section of Scripture is that it goes on to explain what happens when we continue our spiritual walk and what happens to us if we don't.

"The more you grow like this, the more productive and useful you will be in your knowledge of our Lord Jesus Christ." 2 Peter 1:8

As we continue to work a program, we become more available in our spiritual walk to reach out to others. We learn how to pray — not just for ourselves but for others and we learn how to serve others better. We develop boldness in our recovery and our faith. We carry messages of healing hope without shame. We share our testimonies and disclose parts of our lives that caused us to feel shame but are now assets instead of defects. As we develop boldness in our faith, we overcome obstacles. People will see a difference in us, that does not appear as prideful, but gives credit and glory to God.

How are you willing to take all of these principles and practices indicated in these verses...

To be more productive? _____

_____

To be more useful? _____

_____

How will these principles of removing decadence from your life help you be more useful in your knowledge of Jesus Christ?

_____

_____

_____

_____

_____

_____

How will sharing this information and developing faith help you be more productive and useful?

_____

_____

_____

_____

_____

_____

How will being more godly and moral help you be more productive and useful?

_____

_____

_____

_____

_____

_____

How are you willing to patiently endure growing in all these areas?

How are you willing to listen to God and carry the message to others who are struggling and rejoice in the good news?

Forgetting to Remember

"But those who fail to develop in this way are shortsighted or blind, forgetting that they have been cleansed from their old sins." 2 Peter 1:9

In verse 9, we see the warning of consequences for those who do not follow the righteous path revealed in verses 4-8. Many of us live for immediate gratification instead of eternal life. We prefer things that are instant instead of long-term. In recovery and our spiritual lives, we experience consequences because:

- We can't control our human desires
- We fall into the world's corruption
- We don't respond to God's promises
- We don't want to look at our morals
- We don't continue to explore or deepen our faith
- We don't develop our knowledge/wisdom of God, godly people, or God's word
- We don't apply holy actions and Scriptures to our daily lives
- We don't practice self-control
- We are impatient
- We think that attaining godliness is too much work
- We believe that being spiritual is a weakness
- We don't care about our brothers and sisters-only ourselves OR we only care about our brothers and sisters and neglect ourselves
- We don't want to grow up and be productive
- We think that what we learn in a sermon one time per week is enough to know about Jesus

- We take sanctification from sin for granted
- We believe all we need is faith, no works
- We don't want to do all these things and look for a shortcut

From a recovery standpoint:

- We try to find an "easier softer way" (Alcoholics Anonymous Big Book, page 59)
- We don't like some of the steps
- We skip steps
- We think we know better than people who have found recovery
- We think we know better than God
- We didn't "give it away" to keep it
- We don't receive gratification quickly enough from our recovery efforts
- We have been blessed with recovery for such a long time that we forgot what the addiction was like

In recovery, We call this "shortsighted or blind" experience = DENIAL. The acronym for denial is:

Don't

Even

Notice

I

Am

Lying.

We find it strange how many people return to the addictive lifestyle because they think they don't have the problem anymore. They don't realize the reason they don't have the problem anymore is that they were practicing a godly lifestyle! The reason we go to meetings, help newcomers, help set up the meeting and clean up afterward is to remain humble, to help, to remember where we came from, and never to forget that we could end up back in the same place or much worse than we ever imagined.

I used to feel so ashamed of my behaviors and thought I would never get better. I thought I would never get to the point that God could love me. My sins were so overwhelming that I had lost my opportunity for Heaven. Think about that for a minute.

Have you tried to find "Heaven on earth" because you don't think you will be able to go to Heaven? "Live for today" and "you only live once" (yolo) are good sayings for living a good life and trying new things, but not if it's related to destructive behaviors. These are just risks that are detrimental to us and those around us.

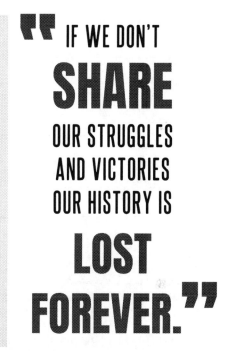

" IF WE DON'T SHARE OUR STRUGGLES AND VICTORIES OUR HISTORY IS LOST FOREVER."

If God has delivered us from harmful behaviors, time causes us to forget what He has done for us. We forget about the pain we experienced in the past. In forgetting, we think we can return to those behaviors again without consequence.

Almost all holidays are to remember the pain that has been relieved and a blessing that has been given. Passover is celebrated to commemorate the suffering of the terrible plagues that Egypt was subjected to as a result of Pharaoh's hard heart and the release of the Hebrew people to freedom. Purim is the feast celebrating the saving of the Jewish people from Haman who planned to kill all the Jewish people in the Persian Empire and the blessing of being able to protect themselves and keep their freedom. Hanukkah is the festival celebrating liberation from oppression, freedom of worship, and finding light in the darkest of times. Christmas is a celebration of the birth of our

Savior, who offers to take away all of our sins. Easter is the celebration of the resurrection of our Savior after being beaten and crucified and being brought back to life-giving everyone an opportunity for eternal life. Other holy days celebrate only the good things, but we can forget those and lose our gratitude and the sacrifices God and others have made for us.

Has there ever been pain or a habit you thought would never return, you dabbled with it, and it took over again?

How long did it take before you are unable to control the habit?

Did you forget to remember those things you told yourself you would never do again?

How many times have we started a relationship with someone that has the same issues as our last relationship?

What old behaviors did you start again, believing that you had control, but found out you didn't?

I frequently ask counseling clients, who have been arrested for multiple DWIs, a simple question, "What are two things that you promised you would never do again after you got your first DWI?" The answer is always "drink and drive. But..."

"But" is an interesting word; it usually erases or attempts to excuse the portion of the sentence that we say before the word "but". We can see an example of this when we look at how 2 Peter 1:8 is erased by verse nine. God presents us with an opportunity that can be "erased" by inattention or losing its significance.

"The more you grow like this, the more productive and useful you will be in your knowledge of our Lord Jesus Christ (Yay!!!). But those who fail to develop in this way are shortsighted or blind, forgetting that they have been cleansed from their old sins." (Awwww...)

If we don't develop these positive characteristics of faith, morals, godliness, etc. we will only live for the moment. We won't see the problems we have and will forget that we were given a reprieve and lost it.

Sometimes people don't want to remember where they came from, but being removed from unfavorable circumstances is a blessing that needs to be announced. It may not have been spectacular, but it is a miracle and a testimony to other people struggling with the same problems or worse.

If we don't share our struggles and victories our history is lost forever.

CHAPTER FIVE

Where would we be if we didn't hear about the struggles and blessings of Job, Joseph, Abraham, Moses, David, Paul, Peter, John, or Jesus? Think about the lessons we learned from each one of their lives. Which two impacted you the most?

_____

_____

_____

_____

_____

_____

_____

_____

_____

_____

Which story from the Bible inspires your recovery, persistence, or endurance?

_____

_____

_____

_____

_____

Who or what have you forgotten that you need to remember to avoid making mistakes?

_____

_____

_____

_____

What have you forgotten that helps you rejoice in victories?

_____

_____

_____

_____

_____

"Works" To Remember Faith

"So, dear brothers and sisters, work hard to prove that you really are among those God has called and chosen. Do these things, and you will never fall away." 2 Peter 1:10

The beauty of verse 10 is: it reminds us that because of His love for us and our faith in Him, we have been allowed to have a new and better life. If we do all that He has asked us, beginning with verse 3, we will never fall away. One of the greatest fears of the person who is in recovery is falling away or falling off the wagon or relapse. There are countless sayings in recovery, but this one reminds us how fragile our lives can be, "I know I have one more relapse in me, but I don't know if I have one more recovery left in me."

One reminder about these verses in 2 Peter, Chapter 1, is that they are not for alcoholics, drug addicts, sex addicts, codependents, overeaters, etc. *THEY ARE FOR SINNERS.*

How many of us are sinners?

These scriptures are for every one of us. We can say that we never saw these before, and we hoped that our spiritual walk would lead us on the path of these virtuous behaviors that develop faith, moral excellence, self-control, patient endurance, godliness, and so on. However, what is essential is that we now have a way to practice these behaviors. The 12-steps give us specific actions to take and ways to live the lifestyle. We have heard family members initially deny there would be any valid reason for them to understand the 12-steps. They often believe that if the person with the sinful behavior will just straighten out their lives, then their lives would be "fixed." One lady responded, after her first codependency meeting, "If everyone knew and lived the 12-steps, the world would be an amazing place."

In the New Testament Scriptures, we are informed that we are saved by grace, not works. But this doesn't mean that some of the things we do for our faith won't take time and effort. At the beginning of our faith, praying, reading the Scriptures, meditating on God's word, going to church, incorporating the word of God into our lives, and being accountable to others will take time and effort. Which one of these things do you need to work on for your life so you can have a better relationship with God?

Are you reading and studying the word? How has reading the Scriptures help your life?

How do you think reading at least one chapter per day would help you?

How much time do you spend with God in prayer?

How do you think fellowshipping with other believers and learning from them and their experiences with God would help your faith?

What are some of the ways you can hear God speaking to you?

Have you ever fallen away from God, your faith, or your church? How did it affect your life?

Who is your spiritual mentor?

How has their input positively impacted your life?

Is there anything that is lacking in your life or anything that you have a difficult time doing regarding prayer, fellowship, reading, or meeting with a mentor?

_____

_____

_____

_____

If you have had a bad experience, how do you think God will provide for the spiritual needs that he encourages you to develop?

_____

_____

_____

_____

Is there anyone you can call that might be able to help you?

_____

_____

_____

_____

Would you be willing to participate in Celebrate Recovery, Stephen's Ministry, or counseling ministries and ask for support?

_____

_____

_____

_____

Obedience Provides a Blessing

"Then God will give you a grand entrance into the eternal Kingdom of our Lord and Savior Jesus Christ." 2 Peter 1:11

Verse 11 reiterates the blessings and promises of serving God ("do these things and you will never fall away"). However, salvation and accepting Christ as our Savior is what allows us to enter the Kingdom of God. Recovery/faith will help us find the path. Doing both of these can provide us with an opportunity to hear those words from God, "Well done my good and faithful servant." God appreciates servants who are productive, useful, knowledgeable, obedient, and glorify Him. The beautiful thing about the next section of verses is that it is titled:

PAYING ATTENTION TO SCRIPTURE
(this is the title of the section in The Life Recovery Bible,
New Living Translation, 2 Peter beginning with verse 12)

"Therefore, I will always remind you about these things—even though you already know them and are standing firm in the truth you have been taught."

In verse 12, Peter tells us that he will always remind us about the positive attributes that Jesus practiced and wants us to practice. All of these virtues were planted in our being as made evident in Psalm 40:8 (NLT), *"I take joy in doing your will, my God, for your instructions are written on my heart"*. We already knew about them; we were just distracted by our desires and pleasures. We have been taught these things in school, in church, and by our parents. As with previous generations, we may have been taught them in Boy Scouts, Girl Scouts, the military or other foundational centers that provide us with values and morals. However, it seems like the modern thought does not tend to teach these values and some people have a hard time identifying with these statements.

Before entering the holy land and after God's people received the Ten Commandments these instructions were given to connect to God and to treat to each other reverently. God told His people this:

"⁹ The LORD your God will then make you successful in everything you do. He will give you many children and numerous livestock, and He will cause your fields to produce abundant harvests, for the LORD will again delight in being good to you as He was to your ancestors. ¹⁰ The LORD your God will delight in you if you obey His voice and keep the commands and decrees written in this Book of Instruction, and if you turn to the LORD your God with all your heart and soul. ¹¹ This command I am giving you today is not too difficult for you, and it is not beyond your reach. ¹² It is not kept in Heaven, so distant that you must ask, 'Who will go up to Heaven and bring it down so we can hear it and obey?' ¹³ It is not kept beyond the sea, so far away that you must ask, 'Who will cross the sea to bring it to us so we can hear it and obey?' ¹⁴ No, the message is very close at hand; it is on your lips and in your heart so that

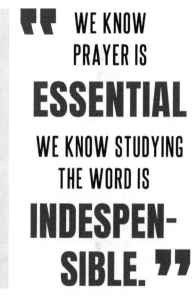

" WE KNOW PRAYER IS **ESSENTIAL** WE KNOW STUDYING THE WORD IS **INDESPEN-SIBLE.** "

you can obey it. ¹⁵ Now listen! Today I am giving you a choice between life and death, between prosperity and disaster. ¹⁶ For I command you this day to love the LORD your God and to keep His commands, decrees, and regulations by walking in His ways. If you do this, you will live and multiply, and the LORD your God will bless you and the land you are about to enter and occupy."
Deuteronomy 30:9-16

I love this Scripture from Deuteronomy. It is a 3000-year-old reminder to God's people that obedience results in blessing. It is a reminder that living a godly life keeps God on our lips and in our hearts so we can live in peace. It's a reminder that God is within us and not far from us. It lets us know that his word is not "too difficult" for us to understand and it is not out of our reach. This reminder is an instruction to love God, follow his commands, decrees, and regulations by living the life He wants us to live. This again is one of those promises discussed in 2 Peter 1:4.

The Alcoholics Anonymous big book has a similar insight.

"Actually, we were fooling ourselves, for deep down in every man, woman, and child, is the fundamental idea of God. It may be obscured by calamity, by pomp, by worship of other things, but in some form or other it is there. For faith in a Power greater than ourselves, and miraculous demonstrations of that power in human lives, are facts as old as man himself.

We finally saw that faith in some kind of God was a part of our make-up, just as much as the feeling we have for a friend. Sometimes we had to search fearlessly, but He was there. He was as much a fact as we were. We found the Great Reality deep down within us. In the last analysis it is only there that He may be found. It was so with us."

Alcoholics Anonymous Big Book, Page 55

We now know what God expects from us. We know prayer is essential, we know studying the word is indispensable, we know that loving our brothers and sisters is required and even fellowshipping with other believers is vital. But, the flesh, earthly desires, cravings, addictions, power, and desire for control will cripple us, causing us to prioritize the world and what it offers over God and what He offers. If we don't know what God wants from us, it is our responsibility to find out. We can choose to learn or ignore what God has put before us. We can learn from elders in the church or the mistakes of brand-new people coming in and seeking help.

Doug was a person new to recovery, who had a strong history of faith. He told me how he overcame his dislike and concerns of the Ten Commandments. He stated, "I realized the Ten

Commandments weren't created to deprive me of enjoyable things in life, but rather to protect me. I choose to call them the 'Ten Don't Hurt Yourselves.'"

When you became a Christian, did you believe that you only had to go to church one time? Why?

_____

_____

_____

Do you think you'll need to open up the Bible only when the pastor does? Why?

_____

_____

_____

Many of us live in a world where we can eat fast food any time, fruit and vegetables are available to us during all seasons and we can eat more than 3 meals per day. Why do you need to pray for food /your daily bread?

_____

_____

_____

_____

Do you only pray when you have problems? If the God of the universe wants a relationship with you, do you think He'd be happy if He only spoke to you when you were in trouble?

_____

_____

_____

_____

CHAPTER FIVE

Why would He want to hear victories, success, and Thanksgiving from you and speak to you all the time?

When you talk to your friends, do you want to be there for them through the good and the bad times?

When you became a Christian, did you stop sinning?

How long do you plan on being a Christian?

Is being a Christian about religion and rules? Or is it about a relationship with Jesus Christ?

Is it worthwhile for you to stay in constant contact with your Creator, so you can be strengthened and renewed? Or should you wait until things really get bad and you need Him to help pick up the pieces that you've neglected?

_____

_____

_____

Can a relationship be maintained with a friend who only calls you when they need you?

_____

_____

_____

How do you feel knowing that obeying and glorifying God "will give you a grand entrance into the eternal Kingdom of our Lord and Savior Jesus Christ"? I look forward to seeing you there!

_____

_____

_____

_____

_____

_____

How Long Do We Have to Do This?

"And it is only right that I should keep on reminding you as long as I live." 2 Peter 1:13

If I have a medical condition like diabetes, do I need to be reminded every day to check my blood sugar levels? Do I need to be reminded to avoid sugar and high-carb foods? Do I need to be retold to do my insulin injection? If I had cancer do I need to be reminded to get quarterly or annual checkups? Do I need to be urged to stay out of the sun if I had skin cancer? If I am a Christian, do I need to be reminded to go to church every Sunday? Do I need to be reminded to read the Scriptures? Do I need to be reminded to pray and thank God for delivering me from my old life? If I have never been able to abstain from my addictive behaviors in the past but found a way to overcome them through recovery, should I continue to attend the meetings? Work the 12-steps? Contact my sponsor? Pray? Meditate? Read and learn about my addiction? Of course, the answer to all of these is a resounding "Yes!"

Well, it turns out that we do need reminders! I have known professionals who have died when their addictions or diseases resurfaced as a result of neglecting recovery practices. I have seen people take their sobriety for granted. They believed they were cured, got bored with recovery, moved to a new town, and pretended like they never had a problem or isolated themselves. Even though we are reminded regularly, we have found it necessary to keep reminding each other as long as we live.

One of the most wonderful experiences we have when helping people find recovery from various problems occurs when we ask what they have learned. Groups of recovering people with a year or more of recovery were asked, "What has been the best part or greatest blessing of recovery?" Almost all of them responded, "We have a real relationship with God now."

The Holy Spirit works to develop the fruit in our lives and helps us grow in grace. We are not doing it alone; God is also working within us. We can look at the thousands of chapters and verses in the Scriptures and be overwhelmed by the daunting task of living how God hopes we will live. The truth is, if we could do it by ourselves, we wouldn't need God. The more we practice these lifestyles, the easier it becomes. We need to work together with God and His people, so we can let God lead us to a spiritual life and recover from this world.

We hope that you can find the same opportunities that we have discovered. We hope that you practice them with others, that you share your experiences with the newcomers, find new ways to love your brothers and sisters and stay close to God for as long as you live.

So, how long should you attend church once you get saved?

_____

_____

How long should you participate in recovery?

_____

_____

When should you stop reading the Scriptures or spiritual writings, stop attending fellowship, and stop living by the teachings of God?

_____

_____

Second Peter was written after Peter relapsed in his faith and then experienced a renewal through his healing process with Jesus and the Holy Spirit. The relapse happened when Peter professed his total commitment to Jesus and his willingness to stay by Jesus' side no matter what anyone else does. (Mark 14:29). Our human nature combined with compulsive behaviors or sinful habits make it hard for us to keep our promises. This is part of our denial of our powerlessness and its effect on our lives. This is what we experience when we work Step 1 by ourselves and without God.

Peter denies Jesus three different times, as Jesus predicted, and resulted in Peter breaking down and crying (Mark 14:72). John went to the crucifixion, but Peter did not. On the third day, when Peter heard the news that Jesus was not in the tomb, he and a few other disciples ran to find the tomb empty and the linen cloth lying in the tomb. The pain that he felt was reduced by the good news that Jesus was alive. Peace and sanity returned and God revealed the power to resurrect and restore Jesus and other people's lives. The disciples were relieved and lucidity resumed. This is what we experience when we work on Step 2.

Peter felt relieved when he heard the news that Mary Magdalene, Joanna, and Mary the mother of James were told that the crucified Jesus has risen from the dead. Peter was specifically named by the angel when he said "tell the disciples, _including Peter_ that they would see Jesus in Galilee" in Mark 16:7. Two of Jesus' followers that were on the road to Emmaus told the 11 disciples that Jesus had appeared to Peter (Luke 24:34). This is the joy we find in Step 3 when we are willing to do whatever God tells us to do and turn our lives over to God.

In Luke 24: 47-48, Jesus lets the disciples know that there is forgiveness for all sins for all who repent. We experience this when we do steps 4 & 5 by confessing to God and others about all of our sins.

Jesus promises to send the Holy Spirit in Luke 24:49 "And now I will send the Holy Spirit, just as my Father promised. But stay here in the city until the Holy Spirit comes and fills you with power from heaven." We have learned what we need to do, but we have a difficult time stopping the bad things and starting to practice what God wants us to do. When we get rid of the evil spirits in our lives, God sends the Holy Spirit to fill us with godly wisdom. This is what we seek and experience when we do Steps 6 and 7.

When Peter and Jesus talk, Jesus asked three times if Peter loves Him. Jesus forgives Peter when he tells Jesus of his love for him and is urged by Jesus to teach, feed, and take care of His sheep. Also that God had examined his ways and forgiven him. Peter confesses brotherly love to Jesus, is humbled and willing to do whatever the Lord said (John 21:18). Making amends and living a godly life (Steps 8 through 10) will be difficult for us, but we're blessed to serve the Lord and glorify God in all we do.

Peter, John, and the other disciples were being taught by Jesus for 40 days before he ascended to heaven (Acts 1:1-3). During the forty days **after** Jesus suffered and died, He appeared to the apostles from time to time and showed them in many ways that he was actually alive. He also spoke to them about the Kingdom of God. This is the blessing of Step 11 when we pray for God's wisdom and guidance and meditate on his word.

Following instructions from Jesus and the angels in Acts 1:8, Jesus tells the disciples they will receive power when the Holy Spirit fills them and will be his witnesses, *"telling people about me everywhere—in Jerusalem, throughout Judea, in Samaria, and to the ends of the earth."* This is what we receive and gladly share when we overcome our destructive habits and have the joy of serving God. This is the great commission described in the last chapter of Matthew and in the last step of the 12-steps.

We are emboldened with changed lives, power from God, reconnecting to our faith, sharing our miracles, and helping whoever, wherever we can, whenever we can.

Thank you for looking at 2 Peter and the journey to finding a stronger relationship with God. I hope you find recovery from whatever unhealthy habit or past hurt is causing separation and pain in your life. I pray that you let go of the false idols and hold on tightly to the one true God.

In the next book, we will review John and follow his guidance for continued recovery.

Printed in the United States
by Baker & Taylor Publisher Services